How to
Develop and Manage

QUALIFICATION
PROTOCOLS
FOR
FDA COMPLIANCE

■ ■ ■

Phil Cloud

informa
healthcare

New York London

First published in 1999 by CRC Press LLC, 2000 N.W. Corporate Blvd., Boca Raton, FL 33431, USA.

This edition published in 2010 by Informa Healthcare, Telephone House, 69-77 Paul Street, London EC2A 4LQ, UK.

Simultaneously published in the USA by Informa Healthcare, 52 Vanderbilt Avenue, 7th Floor, New York, NY 10017, USA.

Informa Healthcare is a trading division of Informa UK Ltd. Registered Office: 37–41 Mortimer Street, London W1T 3JH, UK. Registered in England and Wales number 1072954.

A CIP record for this book is available from the British Library.

Library of Congress Cataloging-in-Publication Data available on application

ISBN-13: 9781574910988

Orders may be sent to: Informa Healthcare, Sheepen Place, Colchester, Essex CO3 3LP, UK
Telephone: +44 (0)20 7017 5540
Email: CSDhealthcarebooks@informa.com
Website: http://informahealthcarebooks.com/

For corporate sales please contact: CorporateBooksIHC@informa.com
For foreign rights please contact: RightsIHC@informa.com
For reprint permissions please contact: PermissionsIHC@informa.com

Contents

Preface

Are you ready for validation? FDA is. FDA regulations, such as current Good Manufacturing Practice (cGMP) for pharmaceuticals, Good Laboratory Practice (GLP), and Good Clinical Practice (GCP), as well as industry standard ISO 9000 require that validation documentation such as qualification protocols be established and followed. But these regulations do not provide guidelines on how to produce the documentation. Individual companies are left to develop their own validation documentation. *How to Develop and Manage Qualification Protocols for FDA Compliance* explains how to develop and manage qualification protocols and their associated documentation for all of the functions of a validation department: cleaning, facilities and utilities, equipment, computers and software, and process. It explains the following:

How to develop equipment and protocol master lists

How to assign identification numbers and names

How to develop protocol formats and style guides

How to establish a documentation review and approval system

How to perform qualification testing

How to write final reports

How to design conditional release and certification forms

How to establish a baseline management system for documentation

How to establish a change control program

How to establish a requal program

How to establish a document control system

How to establish a forms control program

How to change over your documentation system from paper to electronic

How the documents relate to each other and to an overall documentation system

This book also provides hands-on techniques for writing qualification protocols to achieve FDA compliance. Designed for individuals responsible for writing qualification protocols for drug products and related industries, such as drug devices and diagnostics, pharmaceutical biotechnology, and bulk pharmaceutical chemicals, it provides actual examples of protocols,

ix

requal protocols, final reports, certifications, deviations, deficiencies, and addendums, thus anticipating many of your validation documentation questions.

The overall intention of this book is to familiarize you with the essential elements and concepts of qualification protocol development and management and how to apply these concepts to your own validation programs. Validation principles and tools common to all validation functions are emphasized. Step-by-step procedures are shown for protocol formats and contents, with diagrams and other graphics to illustrate key ideas. The book should be useful for all validation practitioners, whether beginning or advanced. Directors, managers, and supervisors of validation staff as well as individuals interested in improving the efficiency of their own validation efforts also may find this book valuable.

My experience with such regulators as FDA, FAA, NASA, and EF&T influenced my decision to write this book. Because regulators do not provide information on how to do things the need for such a book was clear. I am a practitioner of equipment validation, so most of the examples in this book are equipment related, but you will find that they serve to illustrate and explain all kinds of validation.

Phil Cloud

The methods described in this book are those of the author and are not to be construed as the policy of his employer.

Chapter 1

Introduction

This guidebook consists of 35 validation procedures and 30 forms that can be used by old or new and small or large companies to establish a validation documentation system (Fig. 1.1). All of the methods shown in this book should be tailored to fit each company's unique operation. It is written in such a way that it can be used as a guideline by employees who are responsible for writing and managing qualification protocols. The protocol formats and numbering systems can be used by most companies, and they are acceptable to the Food and Drug Administration (FDA). The table of contents follows the normal sequence of a validation process and its documentation. Documentation methods are established in each of the chapters. Several of the procedures include forms that will aid in the information gathering process.

The validation documentation system is the main focus of any validation effort, and it controls the framework of the entire process. Qualification documentation must be developed and approved, prior to use, if it is directly related to the quality, purity, identity, or strength of a product. The challenge today is to perform validation in the most effective and efficient way possible. This book provides a step in that direction.

ORGANIZATION

The simplest method of organizing the validation effort is to divide it up into a logical order, such as cleaning, facilities, utilities, equipment, computer and software, and process (Fig. 1.2). Any combination of related functions is acceptable. For example, equipment and computer can be combined because there are overlapping functions; facilities and utilities can be combined because they are related. Some companies are large enough to have all of the validation functions, but in smaller companies just one person may perform all of the functions. The methods

Figure 1.1   *Validation Documentation System*

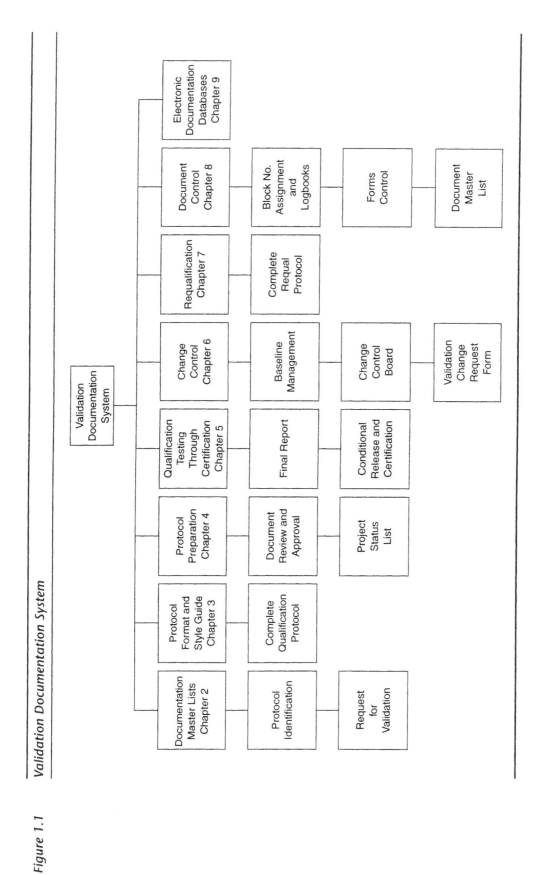

Figure 1.2 **Validation Department Functions**

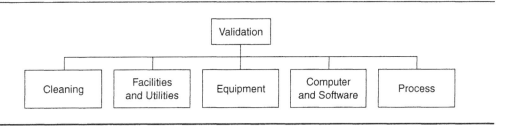

described in this book apply to all of the validation department functions: cleaning, facilities, utilities, equipment, computer and software, and process. I will be using the validation department functions as a means of identifying and organizing validation documentation. Separating the documentation into department functions allows for establishing protocol spreadsheets. The department function's are grouped next to each other for planning purposes. (See Chapter 2 under "Protocol Master List" and Chapter 8 under "Document Master List".)

A VALIDATION STORY

Once upon a time there was a pharmaceutical company that was manufacturing tablets and capsules long before FDA regulations ever existed. When the FDA regulations came into being, the company started validating their manufacturing processes. The formulation of raw materials is where the drug product's strength, quality, and purity are controlled and the company wanted to make sure that they were in compliance and that their products were safe. Next they started validating the equipment that made contact with the product. Eventually they started validating their cleaning processes, facilities, utilities, and computer systems. They formed a validation department and split it up into different validation functions. People were hired; a validation plan, policies, and SOPs were written; and protocol formats were developed. This is where this book comes in. It covers everything it takes to develop and manage qualification protocol documentation.

VALIDATION ELEMENTS

The following list assumes that a company is starting a validation department from scratch. If the validation department already exists, compare this list with your own to see if all the bases have been covered. The complete validation structure has been listed to show the position of this book within a complete validation scheme.

- Set up a validation department

- Write a validation plan

- Write policies, SOPs, and administrative procedures

(Book starts here)

- Identify which system needs to be validated and establish a master list

- Assign protocol writing tasks for each of the validation functions cleaning, facilities, utilities, equipment, computer, software, and process
- Identify critical equipment to validate first, then most important to less important
- Assign equipment numbers
- Assign protocol numbers
- Write and execute qualification protocols
- Establish document reviewers and approvers
- Establish document distribution
- Establish a Change Control Board
- Assign change control numbers
- Change protocols
- Deviations
- Deficiencies
- Addendums
- Requalification
- Document Control

(Book ends here)

- Perform commissioning at the original equipment manufacturer (OEM)
- Internal audits
- FDA audits

VALIDATION DOCUMENTATION

Following are the key validation documents that are developed and retained to support the previously listed validation efforts. This documentation is required to operate and function as a validation department. Only qualification and requalification protocols are covered in this book (Fig. 1.3). Protocols will need to be developed for each of the validation department functions (see Fig. 1.2).

Figure 1.3   **Validation Documentation**

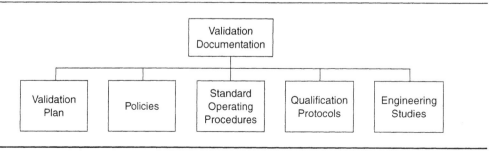

PROTOCOL DOCUMENTATION

All completed qualification and requalification protocols that reside in Document Control shall have a complete set of validation documentation: a protocol package contents sheet, certification form, final report, protocol, deficiency forms (if any), and addendums (if any). Appendix D contains a complete set of all of the required qualification protocol documents shown in Fig. 1.4. They are listed in the order that they should be in when the protocol package is filed in Document Control.

VALIDATION DOCUMENTATION MANAGEMENT

This book shows how to develop and manage qualification protocols and their associated documentation for all validation department functions: cleaning, facilities and utilities, equipment, computer and software, and process. The book is written in the order that validation functions are carried out. First you have to develop equipment and protocol master lists and databases and assign identification numbers and names. Next you will need to develop protocol and form formats and style guides and include tips on how to write protocols and final reports. You will also need to develop a documentation review and approval system.

After you have established the above documentation system you will have the tools in place to record your qualification testing. After qualification testing is complete and approved you will need to develop certification forms and/or execute conditional releases of the equipment.

After the equipment is certified for use you will need to file the validation documentation in Document Control to establish a baseline for your qualification testing. Next you will have to develop a change control system comprised of equipment changes and a requal program.

BASIC PROTOCOL DOCUMENTATION STEPS

The following list is in the order that validation is carried out. It shows what you need to be thinking about as you form your protocol documentation system. The elements shown will keep coming up all the time, therefore, you will need to have a system in place to manage them.

Figure 1.4   **Qualification Protocol Documentation**

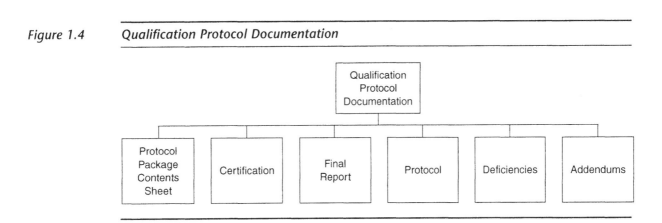

New or requal protocols are written

  Departments

    Review protocols

    Changes are made

  Validation Change Control Board

    Reviews protocol

    Approves

  Qual or requal testing is performed

  Final report is written

  Certifications are issued

  Validation documentation is released into Document Control

  A documentation baseline is established

Qualification protocols are changed

  Departments

    Review

    Changes are made

  Validation Change Control Board

    Reviews

    Approves

  Qual or requal testing is performed (if required)

  Final report is written

  Certifications are issued

  Validation documentation is released into Document Control

  A documentation baseline is established

PROTOCOL WRITING

The protocol writing methods described in this book are designed to support the current Good Manufacturing Practices (cGMP) in a solid dosage from manufacturing environment, but they can be applied to related industries, such as drug device and diagnostics, pharmaceutical biotechnology, and bulk pharmaceutical chemicals. This book provides hands-on techniques for writing qualification and requalification protocols to achieve FDA compliance and includes actual examples of protocols, final reports, certifications, deficiencies, and addendums to provide answers to many of your validation documentation questions. Readers will have a general understanding of validation principles and how to apply these principles in a GMP facility. Simple diagrams and other graphics illustrate key ideas.

The intent of this book is to familiarize the reader with the essential elements and concepts of qualification protocol writing and management and how to apply these concepts to their own specific application. Emphasis will be placed on validation principles and tools that are common to all validation functions, with examples for their use. Step-by-step procedures are shown, with protocol formats, contents, and diagrams that will enable readers to apply these approaches to their own validation programs.

HOW TO USE THIS BOOK

This book covers qualification protocol development and management of all of the processes used in a solid dosage form pharmaceutical manufacturing company. This book can be used in several ways. For example, when preparing to validate a system, such as a piece of equipment or a process, you can look in the appendices A–F under the qualification protocol type for an example protocol. Next you can tailor these protocols to fit your unique validation situation. Because the templates are already filled, you are given concrete examples of how to write qualification protocols and perform the qualification testing. If you have a subject in mind, such as change control, you can go to the table of contents, or, for a more detailed explanation of the subject, use the index. This book can be used for developing and managing validation documentation and for training new employees or retraining existing employees.

Chapter 2

Documentation Master Lists

This chapter covers the first step in the validation process, establishing documentation master lists. The methods described in this chapter apply to all of the validation department functions: cleaning, facilities, utilities, equipment, computer, software, and process. At the beginning of a validation program you will need to establish an equipment master list and then a protocol master list (Fig. 2.1). Spreadsheets can be used for managing these lists. The equipment master list contains the minor, major, and validation-not-required equipment. The protocol master list contains the qualification and requalification protocols for each of the validation department functions. Document number assignment logbooks must be developed and used to provide a method of assigning identification number to all validation documentation. (See Chapter 8 under "Logbooks"). A method for departments outside the validation department to request validation of their systems is also required.

EQUIPMENT MASTER LIST

You will need to identify which systems need to be validated and establish equipment master lists of all of the minor and major equipment and equipment that does not need to be validated. These lists can be developed and changed using spreadsheet software. The validation department will develop a spreadsheet at the startup of a new validation program. You will be using this list daily for planning and scheduling purposes and to answer the big question "Is that piece of equipment validated?" You will be asked this question all the time by the equipment users and the FDA. It is best to have all of the equipment categories on the same master list for instant answers. The equipment master list will capture the following information: equipment number, serial number, equipment description, equipment location, and whether validation is required. The following paragraphs explain how to assign equipment numbers and names.

Figure 2.1   **Documentation Master Lists**

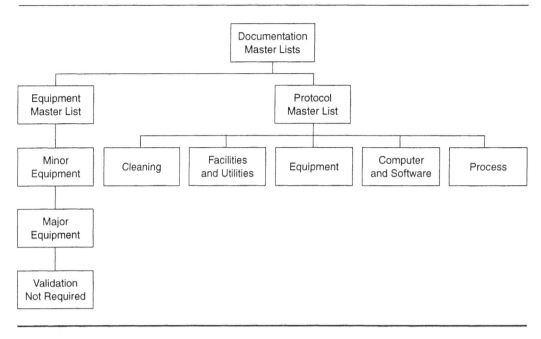

Table 2.1   **Minor Equipment List**

Equipment Number	Serial Number	Description	Location/ Room	Reason Not Validated
01	128507	Groen Steam Kettle	215	N/A
02	128510	Groen Steam Kettle	216	N/A
03	8537	C. E. Tyler Rotap Sieve Shaker	211	N/A
04	8547	C. E. Tyler Rotap Sieve Shaker	212	N/A
Etc.				

The above list is just a portion of the complete equipment master list.

Equipment Numbering System

The equipment number is usually the asset number assigned by the bean counters (accounting department). Tables 2.1 through 2.3 show the methods used to establish equipment numbers— that is, if you have a say in how they are developed. Intelligence or the equipment's description is not needed in the identification number because you will be sorting the list by the description, not the number. The only intelligence that I have in the number is its length. The length of the number distinguishes between minor or major equipment and equipment not validated. Because most spreadsheets are left-justified, zeros have been added to the left of the numbers so that when you sort by the numbers everything is lined up.

- A two-digit number indicates that the equipment is a minor piece of equipment. This method allows for 99 pieces of minor equipment (Table 2.1).

Table 2.2   **Major Equipment List**

Equipment Number	Serial Number	Description	Location/ Room	Reason Not Validated
001	82-6490	Fette Model 2090 Tablet Press	Dev Lab	N/A
002	09-066	Fette Model 3090 Tablet Press	Dev Lab	N/A
003	12A289	34 Station Manesty Unipress Tablet Press	743	N/A
004	I661396	Stokes RD-3 (D) Tablet Press	652	N/A
Etc.				

The above list is just a portion of the complete equipment master list.

Table 2.3   **Validation-Not-Required List**

Equipment Number	Serial Number	Description	Location/ Room	Reason Not Validated
001	82-6490	Fette Model 2090 Tablet Press	Dev Lab	N/A
0001	P32739	Mettler Model AE10 Precision Balance	Dev Lab	Calibrated
0002	B56943	Mettler Model AE100 Precision Balance	Dev Lab	Calibrated
0003	G86126	Sartorious Model IP65 Balance	Dev Lab	Calibrated
0004	15311	Talboy Model 134-2 T-line Stirrer	Dev Lab	Utensil
Etc.				

The above list is just a portion of the complete equipment master list.

- A three-digit number indicates that the equipment is a major piece of equipment. This method allows for 999 pieces of major equipment (Table 2.2).

- A four-digit number indicates that the equipment does not need to be validated. This method allows for 9,999 pieces of equipment that do not need to be validated (Table 2.3).

Equipment Description

The equipment description will need to follow a set pattern, such as: Fette Model 2090 Tablet Press. This is called the noun phrase method—the noun being "tablet press" and the phrase being the manufacturer's name and model number and/or any other identifying information so that you can distinguish between different pieces of equipment. If several pieces of equipment have the same description, the serial number will help identify which is which. The serial number is assigned by the equipment manufacturer and is usually found on the equipment or in the literature that is sent along with the equipment.

Minor Equipment

Deciding if a piece of equipment is minor or major is not an exact science. Table 2.1 shows some examples of minor equipment. One distinction is that minor equipment is not used to manufacture the end product. It usually provides a supporting role to major equipment. An example would be a drum stirring mixer that stirs the coating materials prior to the tablet coating process. The tablet coating pan is the major equipment, and the drum stirring mixer is the minor equipment. Another example would be, after tablets are produced, a hardness tester is used to measure the hardness of a tablet. The tablet press is the major equipment, and the hardness tester is the minor equipment.

Minor equipment is used in support of major equipment. Table 2.1 shows an example of minor equipment. The minor equipment list is just a portion of the complete equipment master list.

Major Equipment

Major equipment is used to manufacture the end product. Table 2.2 shows an example of major equipment. The major equipment list is just a portion of the complete equipment master list.

Validation Not Required Equipment

A few words are needed about equipment that does not need to be validated, because invariably somebody will ask, "Is that piece of equipment validated?" It is always good to explain why the equipment is not validated on the master list. Therefore, when asked why something is not validated, you can look it up in the master list to quickly find the answer. Table 2.3 shows an example of equipment that does not need to be validated. The validation not required list is just a portion of the complete equipment master list.

The types of equipment that do not need to be validated are:

- Calibrated equipment: The complete piece of equipment is designed in such a way that the whole piece of equipment is calibrated, such as a balance or a scale. For example, a large piece of equipment where some of the instruments are calibrated will still need to be validated and the calibrated instruments will be noted in the protocol.

- Utensil: A device that has no control specifications and no measurements. An example would be a device that replaces what an operator would do by hand (i.e., stir plates, stir rods, and spatulas). Glassware that is used to measure a volume is certified and sometimes calibrated by the vendor.

- Instrument: A device that takes a physical measurement and displays a value, but has no control or analytical function (i.e., stopwatches, timers, and thermometers).

Complete Equipment Master List

Following is a combined list of all of the above types of equipment. You can see that the length of the number automatically sorts the equipment into major, minor, and validation not required categories. Equipment numbers that appear in the complete equipment master list are assigned from the equipment number assignment logbooks in Chapter 8. This list answers the following questions:

- What is the equipment number?

- What is the serial number?

- What is the description of the equipment?

- What is the location of the equipment at the time of validation?

- Is the equipment validated?

℞		Equipment Master List		
Equipment Number	Serial Number	Description	Location /Room	Reason Not Validated
❶	❷	❸	❹	❺

Equipment Master List Preparation

Each of the following circled numbers corresponds to the circled number on the equipment master list.

❶ Equipment Number: Enter the next available equipment number from the equipment number assignment log. (See Chapter 8 under "Equipment Number Assignment Log".)

Example: 00, 000, or 0000

❷ Serial Number: Enter the serial number of the equipment.

Example: B56943

❸ Description: Enter the description of the equipment.

*Example:*Talboy Model 134-2 T-line Stirrer (See Page 28 under "Equipment Description".)

❹ Location/Room: Enter the location of the equipment at the time of validation.

❺ Equipment Validated?: Enter yes or no or the reason why the equipment is not validated.

Example: Calibrated, utensil, or instrument

Completed Equipment Master List

This list is sorted off of the equipment number to show how the different length of numbers.

EQUIPMENT NUMBER ASSIGNMENT

The numbering system in this part of the book is for manual paperbased documentation systems. In the paperbased system you will need logbooks to record your documentation numbers. Using logbooks allows you to see what the next available number is when you need to assign a new number. There needs to be a logbook in Document Control where equipment numbers are assigned. (See Chapter 8 under "Equipment Number Assignment Log.")

PROTOCOL MASTER LIST

After you have developed the equipment master list, you should identify which protocols need to be written and establish a qualification and requal protocol master list. The list will show all the protocol numbers that have been assigned. This is the key listing used for planning, scheduling, and status of all validation projects. The protocol master list is used for identifying the latest protocol number assigned for each type of system. The protocol master list will cover all of the validation department functions-cleaning, facilities, utilities, equipment, computer, software, and process. This list will answer the following questions:

- What is the qualification or requalification protocol number?
- What is the description of the document?
- What is the equipment number (if any)?
- What is the serial number (if applicable)?
- What is the location of the equipment at the time of validation (if applicable)?
- Who produced the document?
- When was the document completed?

Ŗ	Equipment Master List				
Equipment Number	Serial Number	Description	Location/ Room	Reason Not Validated	
01	128507	Groen Steam Kettle	215	N/A	
02	128510	Groen Steam Kettle	216	N/A	
03	8537	C. E. Tyler Rotap Sieve Shaker	211	N/A	
04	8547	C. E. Tyler Rotap Sieve Shaker	212	N/A	
001	82-6490	Fette Model 2090 Tablet Press	Dev Lab	N/A	
002	09-066	Fette Model 3090 Tablet Press	Dev Lab	N/A	
003	12A289	34 Station Manesty Unipress Tablet Press	743	N/A	
004	I661396	Stokes RD-3 (D) Tablet Press	652	N/A	
0001	P32739	Mettler Model AE10 Precision Balance	Dev Lab	Calibrated	
0002	B56943	Mettler Model AE100 Precision Balance	Dev Lab	Calibrated	
0003	G86126	Sartorious Model IP65 Balance	Dev Lab	Calibrated	
0004	15311	Talboy Model 134-2 T-line Stirrer	Dev Lab	Utensil	
Etc.					

℞	Protocol Master List					
Protocol Number	Description	Equip. No.	Serial No.	Location /Room	Name	Com. Date
❶	❷	❸	❹	❺	❻	❼

Protocol Master List Preparation

Each circled number below corresponds to the circled number on the example protocol master list.

❶   Protocol Number: Enter the next available protocol or requal protocol number. (See Chapter 8 under "Protocol Number Assignment Log.")

Example: 7006 (process validation new protocol number)

❷   Description: Enter the document description.

Example: (Product Name) USP 600/150 mg, 4 M

❸   Equipment No.: Enter the equipment number, if any.

❹   Serial No.: Enter the serial number, if applicable.

❺   Location/Room: Enter the location of equipment at the time of validation, if applicable.

❻   Name: Enter the name of the person that produced the protocol.

❼   Com. Date: Enter the date when the qual or requal protocols are completed and ready for filing in Document Control.

℞	Protocol Master List					
Protocol Number	Description	Equip. No.	Serial No.	Location /Room	Name	Com. Date
1045	Equipment Cleaning for (Product Name)	-	-	-	PAC	01/24/98
1045 A	Equipment Cleaning for (Product Name)	-	-	-	PAC	03/01/98
2007	Production Room Qualification, Room 147	-	-	Room 147	PAC	02/02/98
3089 B	Distilled Water System, QA Laboratory	125	Y3417	QC Lab	PAC	03/24/98
4009	Compu-Coat 4 Tablet Coating Machine	864	CP001	Room 356	PAC	04/17/98
5023 C	Datamyte Addendum 2, Version 1.1-R&D	534	BM00	Room 479	PAC	05/28/98
6028	AS400 System Software	-	-	-	PAC	06/10/98
7002	(Product Name) USP 300/30 mg, 2.8 M	-	-	-	PAC	7/29/98
Etc.						

Figure 2.2   **Protocol Number Structure**

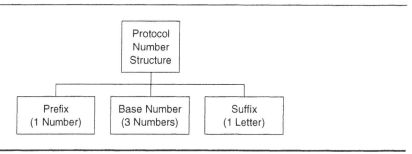

Completed Protocol Master List

This list is sorted off of the protocol number.

PROTOCOL NUMBERING SYSTEM

All qualification and requalification protocols need to have a unique number assigned to them for identification and tracking purposes. The protocol number is used as a locator in a spreadsheet and in Document Control. Fig. 2.2 shows an example of a block numbering system for qualification and requalification protocol numbers. There are two numbering systems shown in this book. This section is for manual paperbased documentation systems and the one in Chapter 9 is for electronic documentation systems.

Qualification and Requalification Protocol Number Structure

This number structure allows you to identify which department the protocol belongs to and uniquely identifies each qualification or requalification protocol. Note the components of the following example protocol number:

4010 C

4 = Prefix

010 = Base number

C = Suffix

Prefix.   The prefix of the protocol number is used to identify each of the validation department functions.

1 = Cleaning

2 = Facilities

3 = Utilities

4 = Equipment

5 = Computer

6 = Software

7 = Process

For example, the 1000 block of numbers is reserved for cleaning validation protocols. The 4-digit numbers allow for 999 different protocol number assignments for each validation department function. Therefore, if you have a 4-digit number that starts with 5, you know that it is a new computer validation protocol. If you have a 4-digit number that starts with 2, you know you have a facilities validation protocol.

Base Number. The three numerical digits following the prefix are the base number of the protocol. This number will be the same for qualification and requalification protocols.

000 to 999 allows for 999 different protocols for each department function

Suffix. The suffix of the protocol number is for requals to the original protocol.

A to Z = 26 requalifications of the original protocol

Example Protocol Numbers and Interpretation

Following are some examples of how to identify a document by its assigned number. The number identifies the department function that is responsible for the protocol, and if this is a new qualification, how many protocols have been written and whether the system has been requaled and how many times. An example of how to use the protocol identification number information is when you need an example of how to develop a new protocol you would not use protocol number 0032 if your numbering system is up to 1450.

Complete Number	Interpretation
3002	This would be the second new utilities protocol that was written.
5055	This would be the 55th new computer protocol written.
4027 H	This would be the eighth requal of the 27th equipment protocol written.

PROTOCOL TITLE

The protocol title is the most important locator because most people remember the title better than the number. You will be naming your protocols so that you can easily identify which system was validated just by reading the title. The protocol title will be the same as the systems description plus a few modifiers (Table 2.4). The name will have to follow a set pattern—for equipment it would be "Fette Model 2090 Tablet Press." The model number and/or any other identifying information helps you distinguish between different pieces of equipment. This naming method allows you to group similar systems next to each other in a spreadsheet.

PROTOCOL NUMBER ASSIGNMENT

The numbering system in this part of the book is for manual paperbased documentation systems. In the paperbased system you will need logbooks to record your documentation numbers. Using logbooks allows you to see what the next

Table 2.4	*Titles Sorted in Alphabetical Order*
	Fette Model 2090 Tablet Press
	Fette Model 3090 Tablet Press
	Manesty Unipress 34 Station Tablet Press
	Stokes RD-3 (D) Tablet Press

available number is when you need to assign a new number. There needs to be a logbook in Document Control where protocol numbers are assigned (See Chapter 8 under "Protocol Number Assignment Log"). Chapter 9 shows an electronic method of assigning protocol numbers when you are ready to change over to an electronic documentation system. Imagine this, there are going to be companies that will be starting up in the computer age and they will not have a paperbased documentation system to transition from.

REQUEST FOR VALIDATION

Any department can request validation of their system. This includes cleaning, facilities, utilities, equipment, computer, software, and process functions. The following form allows outside departments a method of requesting validation of their system. When equipment is involved, it will be found and identified by the validation department at the beginning of a validation program, but as you can imagine, it is not easy to find all of them the first time through. Sometimes the equipment is in storage in a warehouse, or it has not been used for years, or new equipment has been purchased.

Request for Validation Form

With this form you will be answering the following questions:

*   Who is requesting the validation?

*   What is the request for validation number?

*   What is the reason for the request?

*   What is the schedule for the validation?

*   What is the equipment's name, model number, equipment number, serial number, and location (if applicable)?

*   Which documents are included with the request package?

*   Was the request accepted or rejected?

*   What qualification testing will be conducted?

*   What priority was assigned to this validation?

*   Who is going to perform the qualification?

*   Who reviewed and approved this request?

Ŗ	**Request for Validation Form**	
Originator: ❶	Date:	RFV No.: ❷

Department:	Extension:

Reason for Validation: ❸

Schedule Information: ❹

Equipment Name: ❺	Manufacturer:
Model Number:	Equipment Number:
Serial Number:	Location:

The following documentation shall be included with this request. (Check all that are included.)

❻

- ❑ Capitol Appropriation Request
- ❑ Quote
- ❑ Purchase Order
- ❑ Invoice

- ❑ Operations & Maintenance Manual
- ❑ Drawings
- ❑ Operation & Cleaning SOPs (can be in draft form)

❑ Accept ❼	❑ Not Required (Explain.)
Testing to be conducted: IQ OQ PQ	
Priority: Routine Urgent	
Validation Specialist:	
Comments:	

Validation Manager Approval: ❽	Date:

Form Number: V001 (5/28/98)   Reference: SOP-VAL001

Request for Validation Form Preparation

Each of the following circled numbers corresponds to the circled number on the example request for validation form.

❶   Originator: Enter your name, date, department number, and phone extension.

❷   RFV No.: Enter the next available request for validation form number. (See Chapter 8 under "Request for Validation Form Number Assignment Log.")

❸   Reason for Validation: Enter the reason validation is required.

❹   Schedule Information: Enter schedule requirements for the validation.

❺   Equipment Name: Enter the equipment's name, manufacturer's name, model number, equipment number, serial number, and the location of the equipment even if portable, if applicable.

❻   Reference Documentation: Mark all of the boxes that apply and then attach copies.

❼   Validation Department: Mark the appropriate box, either "Accept" or "Not Required", then check the type of qualification testing that will be conducted. Indicate priority by checking either "routine" or "urgent"; note the responsible validation specialist who will be performing the qualification testing. If rejected, enter an explanation.

❽   Validation Manager: Enter your name and date upon acceptance.

Ŗ	**Request for Validation Form**		
Originator:		Date:	RFV No.: 001
Department:		Extension:	

Reason for Validation:

This is a new piece of equipment.

Schedule Information:

This validation needs to be completed by the end of the month.

Equipment Name: Friabilator	Manufacturer: Any Friabilator Co.
Model Number: 90801	Equipment Number: 5910
Serial Number: CD48107924	Location: R&D Laboratory

The following documentation shall be included with this request. (Check all that are included.)

❏ Capitol Appropriation Request	⊠ Operations & Maintenance Manual
❏ Quote	⊠ Drawings
⊠ Purchase Order	⊠ Operation & Cleaning SOPs (can be in draft form)
❏ Invoice	

⊠ Accept	❏ Not Required (Explain.)
Testing to be conducted: IQ✓ OQ✓ PQ✓	
Priority: Routine✓ Urgent	
Validation Specialist: Comments: Standard validation methods.	

Validation Manager Approval:	Date:

Form Number: V001 (5/28/98)   Reference: SOP-VAL001

REQUEST FOR VALIDATION FORM NUMBER ASSIGNMENT

There are form numbers and standard operating procedure (SOP) numbers shown at the bottom of the previous form examples. The methods of assigning form numbers is explained in Chapter 8 under "Request for Validation Form Number Assignment Log" and for SOPs under "Forms Control".

Chapter 3

Protocol Format and Style Guide

This chapter covers the next logical step in the validation process, protocol format. The Food and Drug Administration (FDA) has mandated that companies must supply documented evidence providing a high degree of assurance that the equipment does what it is supposed to do and that the process will consistently produce a product that meets its predetermined specifications and quality attributes. The pharmaceutical industry has developed qualification protocols that are used to conform to the mandate. The protocol methods shown in this book apply to all validation department functions. See Appendices A through F for filled-in examples of each type of qualification protocol.

The qualification protocol is the principal document of the validation process. This chapter shows an example of an installation, operational, and performance qualification protocol (Fig. 3.1). The qualification protocol is the industry tool used to document the qualification process, but it could take any form or format. A qualification protocol will need to be developed and approved before qualification testing can begin. During qualification testing, the performer and reviewer will sign the protocol at the bottom of each page where entries are made. The validation is complete when all acceptance criteria have been met. Protocols are test procedures, and when they are executed they become test reports. These reports are snapshots in time and are archived that way, not to be changed.

Protocol attachments are created to allow for the addition of other departments' and companies' documentation, such as test data results, deficiencies and batch records, certifications, etc. The protocol will be written by a validation specialist and approved by the validation manager, Research and Development, Operations, Maintenance, and Regulatory Compliance. Upon approval, the protocol will be used to perform qualification testing, then it will become part of the validation documentation package and placed in Document Control.

The protocol format shown in this chapter is for a new piece of equipment. The same format is used for the requal protocol format (See Chapter 7) with a few

25

Figure 3.1   **Equipment Qualification Protocol Contents**

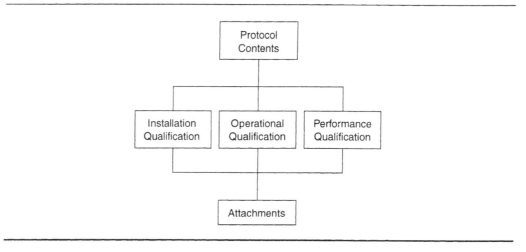

exceptions. The idea is to have all of your information gathering documents the same, as much as possible, because being repetitive is more economical. Any time you have variations in your tasks you waste time and money.

PROTOCOL FORMAT

This chapter will show you how to develop a complete equipment qualification protocol. The method of development applies the same to all validation department functions (all of the other types of protocols are shown in Appendices A through F). You need to capture the most pertinent information that would identify which qualification this is, which equipment is being validated, and who prepared and approved the protocol. With this protocol you will be answering the following questions:

- What is the protocol number?

- Which equipment is being validated?

- Who is the equipment manufacturer?

- What is the model number and the serial number?

- What is the equipment number?

- What was the location of the equipment at the time of testing?

- Who prepared the protocol?

- Who reviewed and approved the protocol?

- Was the qualification testing successful?

Qualification Protocol – Page 1

Following is an example of the first page of an equipment qualification protocol. You need to record the information that identifies the equipment that is being

R̶	Equipment Qualification Protocol		
Title: ❶		Protocol No.: ❷	
Manufacturer: ❸			Page: ❹
Model Number: ❺	Serial Number: ❻		
Equipment Number: ❼	Location: ❽		

Cover Page

❾ Prepared By:	
Validation:	Date:

❿ Approved By:	
Validation Manager:	Date:
Research & Development:	Date:
Operations:	Date:
Maintenance:	Date:
Regulatory Compliance:	Date:

validated, the protocol number, and the page number and the signatures of all applicable reviewers and approvers.

Qualification Protocol – Page 1 Preparation

Each of the following circled numbers corresponds to the circled number on page 1 of the example equipment qualification protocol.

❶   Title: Enter the title. (See Chapter 2 under "Protocol Title.")

Example: (Any Mixer Co.) Model ME501 Emulsifying Mixer

❷   Protocol No.: Enter the protocol number. (See Chapter 8 under "Protocol Number Assignment Log.")

Example: 4010 (equipment validation protocol number)

❸   Manufacturer: Enter the name of the manufacturer.

❹   Page: Enter the page number.

Example: Page 1 of 9.
This method is best for change control purposes because you will need to account for every page of the protocol.

❺   Model Number: Enter the model number.

❻   Serial Number: Enter the serial number.

❼   Equipment Number: Enter the equipment number. (See Chapter 2 under "Equipment Numbering System.")

Example: Minor Equipment Number: 00
         Major Equipment Number: 000

❽   Location: Enter the location of the equipment when it is tested, even if it is portable.

❾   Prepared By: Enter your name and the date when the protocol is complete.

❿   Approved By: Enter your name and the date when your review and approval is complete.

Qualification Protocol – Page 2

Following is an example of the second page of an equipment qualification protocol. You do not need to repeat the entire header on subsequent pages; you only need the information that identifies the equipment being validated, the protocol number, and the page number. Following is an example of a footer for the second page of a qualification protocol. The footer for some of the subsequent pages is different from page 1 because on pages where entries are made, the person who performed the qualification testing will sign and date each page. Also, the person who reviewed the completed protocol will sign and date the protocol. There is nothing at the bottom of the page if entries are not made.

Qualification Protocol – Page 2 Preparation

Each of the following circled numbers corresponds to the circled number on the subsequent pages of the example equipment qualification protocol.

❶   Protocol No.: Enter the protocol number. This is the same number that is on page 1.

❷   Title: Enter the title. This is the same title that is on page 1.

❸   Page Number: Enter the page number.

Example: Page 1 of 9
This method is best for change control purposes because you will need to account for every page of the protocol.

❹   Performed By: The person who performed the test will sign and date here. This footer goes only on the pages where entries are made.

❺   Verified By: The person who reviewed the protocol will sign and date here. This does not necessarily need to be done during qualification testing.

℞ **Equipment Qualification Protocol**	Protocol No.: ❶
Title: ❷	Page: ❸

Subsequent Pages

⤹   This is only on the pages where entries are made.

Performed By: ❹	Date:
Verified By: ❺	Date:

Figure 3.2   ***Equipment Qualification Protocol Elements***

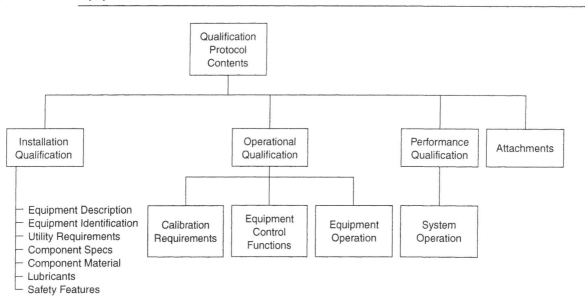

COMPLETE EQUIPMENT QUALIFICATION PROTOCOL

Fig. 3.2 illustrates the major elements of an equipment qualification protocol. The protocol examples in this book can be used as cGMP compliance guides, and they should be tailored to meet individual company requirements. The following pages show examples of completed equipment qualification protocol.

℞	Equipment Qualification Protocol	
Title: (Any Mixer Co.) Model ME501 Emulsifying Mixer		Protocol No.: 4010
Manufacturer: Any Mixer Co.		Page: 1 of 21
Model Number: MC501	Serial Number: 55356 B	
Equipment Number: 2052	Location: Room 802 (This equipment is portable.)	

Prepared By:	
Validation:	Date:
Approved By:	
Validation Manager:	Date:
Research & Development:	Date:
Operations:	Date:
Maintenance:	Date:
Regulatory Compliance:	Date:

Ŗ **Equipment Qualification Protocol**	Protocol No.: 4010
Title: (Any Mixer Co.) Model ME501 Emulsifying Mixer	Page: 2 of 21

Table of Contents

℞ **Equipment Qualification Protocol**	Protocol No.: 4010
Title: (Any Mixer Co.) Model ME501 Emulsifying Mixer	Page: 3 of 21

2.0   Objective

The objective of this equipment qualification is to establish documented evidence that the emulsifying mixer is acceptably installed per manufacturer recommendations, process requirements, and/or engineering standards. Acceptable installation includes suitable utility connections, components, and critical instruments in current calibration. Is fully operational as specified by the protocol. Acceptable operation includes, as applicable, proper control and sequencing functions, recording and reporting functions, and safety and alarm features that meet process requirements and equipment specifications. Acceptable performance includes consistent operation within specified process parameters under simulated or actual production conditions.

3.0   Scope

The scope of this equipment qualification protocol includes the emulsifying mixer and its associated components. Installation qualification is limited to the system components and does not include installation of support utilities, other than the connections at the system boundary. Operational testing is limited to demonstrating equipment functionality. Product specific testing is outside the scope of this qualification document, other than where a product is used to demonstrate equipment functionality.

4.0   Equipment Description

This section will explain how to validate an emulsifying mixer that is motor driven and operates at a fixed speed. All mixing operations are operator controlled with respect to duration and endpoint determination. The mixer provides high shear agitation to moderately low viscosity fluids. As viscosity and/or density increase the volume that the mixer will be able to handle effectively will decrease. The mixer is used in the preparation of solutions for use in a wet granulation process. The mixer cannot be operated without the impeller being submerged in water or other representative fluid or powder.

R Equipment Qualification Protocol	Protocol No.: 4010
Title: (Any Mixer Co.) Model ME501 Emulsifying Mixer	Page: 4 of 21

5.0   Installation Qualification (IQ)

An IQ evaluation will establish confidence that the equipment is properly installed. The installation must meet the manufacturer's specified guidelines along with design changes at installation. Also, the supporting electrical utilities must meet all electrical codes. The information required for an IQ evaluation should be: equipment identification, required documentation, equipment utility requirements, major component specifications, component material, lubricants and equipment safety features.

5.1   Equipment Identification

Record the equipment identification numbers in Table I, along with the following information: equipment manufacturer, purchase order number, model number, serial number, company assigned equipment number, and the location of the equipment.

Writing Tip: The following information is found on the nameplate (placard) attached to the equipment and the equipment manufacturer's installation and operations manual.

Table I   Equipment Identification

Required Information	As-found Conditions
Manufacturer	Any Mixer Co.
Purchase Order Number	004482
Model Number	Series 001 Model MC 501
Serial Number	55356 B
Equipment Number	2052
Location	Room 802 (This equipment is portable.)

Performed By:	Date:
Verified By:	Date:

℞ **Equipment Qualification Protocol**	Protocol No.: 4010

Title: (Any Mixer Co.) Model ME501 Emulsifying Mixer	Page: 5 of 21

5.2   Required Documentation

Record the equipment manufacturer's operation and maintenance manual and drawings in Table II. Record the standard operating procedures that cover the setup, operation and cleaning of the mixer in Table III.

Table II   Required Documentation

Number	Description	Date
None	*Installation Operation Instructions*	*None*
D-1346	*Standard Production Mixer Emulsifier*	*1/4/83*

Table III   Standard Operating Procedures

Number	Description	Release Date
GRA025	Granulation Equipment Setup	10/23/92
GRA026	Granulation Department Equipment Cleaning Procedure	03/12/96

5.3   Equipment Utility Requirements

Compare the manufacturer's specified volt (V) and amps (A) requirements to their as-found condition at the time of qualification testing and record the results in Table IV. Also, record the location of the power supply source. Record the instrument used to measure the volts and amps in Table V.

Performed By:	Date:
Verified By:	Date:

℞ Equipment Qualification Protocol	Protocol No.: 4010
Title: (Any Mixer Co.) Model ME501 Emulsifying Mixer	Page: 6 of 21

Volt Calculation:

Volt specification = 460 V ±10%
±10% of 460 = ±46
460 + 46 = 506
460 - 46 = 414
The measured volts of 461/468/466 fall within ±10%

Amp Calculation:

Circuit rating = 20 A
Equipment current draw = 12.2 A
The circuit amp rating of 20 is greater than the maximum current draw of the equipment

Table IV   Utilities

Utility	Specified	Measured Results	Acceptable (Yes/No)
Volts	460 ±10%	A-B 461 A-C 468 B-C 466	Yes
Amps	Motor = 12.2	20 Circuit Rating	Yes

Power supply source, breaker box BB1, wire numbers: 31, 33, 35.

Table V   Instrument Used

Test Instrument	Identification Number	Calibration Due Date
Multimeter	ME-025	04/19/97

Performed By:		Date:
Verified By:		Date:

R Equipment Qualification Protocol	Protocol No.: 4010
Title: (Any Mixer Co.) Model ME501 Emulsifying Mixer	Page: 7 of 21

5.4 Major Component Specifications

The section is used to verify that the mixer components purchased were delivered and installed. Record the major components in Table VI.

Table VI Major Components

Components	As-found Conditions
Mixer Motor	Manufacturer: Any Motor Co. Model Number: ME 501 Serial Number: 55356 C Volts: 460 Amperes: 12.2 Phases: 3 Cycles: 60 Hz hp: 5 rpm: 3480
Shaft	Part Number: 45267 Size: 1/2" diameter by 36" long Material: 316 Stainless Steel
Impeller	Part Number: 45268 Size: 1/2" bore by 6" diameter Material: 316 Stainless Steel
Performed By:	Date:
Verified By:	Date:

℞ Equipment Qualification Protocol	Protocol No.: 4010
Title: (Any Mixer Co.) Model ME501 Emulsifying Mixer	Page: 8 of 21

5.4   Major Component Specifications

The section is used to verify that the mixer components purchased were delivered and installed. Record the major components in Table VI.

Table VI   Major Components

Components	As-found Conditions
Mixer Motor	Manufacturer: Any Motor Co. Model Number: ME 501 Serial Number: 55356 C Volts: 460 Amperes: 12.2 Phases: 3 Cycles: 60 Hz hp: 5 rpm: 3480
Shaft	Part Number: 45267 Size: 1/2" diameter by 36" long Material: 316 Stainless Steel
Impeller	Part Number: 45268 Size: 1/2" bore by 6" diameter Material: 316 Stainless Steel

Performed By:	Date:
Verified By:	Date:

℞ Equipment Qualification Protocol	Protocol No.: 4010
Title: (Any Mixer Co.) Model ME501 Emulsifying Mixer	Page: 9 of 21

- Never touch a mixer, which has an electric motor, or any part of an electrical service line cord with wet hands or wet feet or if standing on a wet surface.

- Never attempt to move or adjust a mixer while it is running.

- Never touch any rotating part of a mixer with bare hands, gloved hands or with any hand-held object. Rotating parts include, but are not limited to, the mixer shaft, impeller(s), mechanical seals and motor fans.

- Do not touch a mixer motor until it cools. The motor temperature may be high enough to cause burns to the hands.

6.0 Operational Qualification (OQ)

An OQ evaluation should establish that the equipment can operate within specified tolerances and limits. The mechanical ranges of the mixer are being challenged along with the basic mixer operations. The mixer will be validated for its operating ability, not how well it mixes liquids or powders. The information required for the OQ evaluation should be: calibration of the instrument used to control the mixer, equipment control functions (switches and pushbuttons) and equipment operation (mixer rotation direction and mixer speed).

6.1 Calibration Requirements

Verify that all critical instruments on the equipment are logged into the calibration system, have calibration procedures in place and are currently in calibration at the time of qualification testing. Record all of the necessary information for the calibrated instruments used to control the mixer in Table IX.

Performed By:	Date:
Verified By:	Date:

℞　Equipment Qualification Protocol	Protocol No.: 4010
Title: (Any Mixer Co.) Model ME501 Emulsifying Mixer	Page: 10 of 21

Table IX　Calibrated and Non Calibrated Instruments

There were no calibrated or non calibrated instruments on this equipment.

Instrument	As-found Conditions
None	

6.2　Equipment Control Functions

Test Objective. The objective of this test is to verify that the switches on the mixer operate per manufacturer specifications. The mixer will be operated with the impeller submerged in water. The controls that need to be tested are: On Switch and Off Switch.

Test Procedure.

Materials and instruments required: mixing container, test fluid

- Fill the mixing container with water to its maximum working volume of 103 L and record the amount used in Table X. When operating the mixer the head must be submerged in the water to prevent damage to the mixer.

Test Fluid Volume Calculation:

Test fluid volume = 75% of 138 L = 103.5 L (rounded off to 103 L)

- Press the On Switch and verify that the mixer starts operating then record the results in Table XI.

Performed By:	Date:
Verified By:	Date:

℞ Equipment Qualification Protocol	Protocol No.: 4010	
Title: (Any Mixer Co.) Model ME501 Emulsifying Mixer		Page: 11 of 21

- Press the Off Switch and verify that the mixer stops operating then record the results in Table XI.

Table X   Test Materials

Item	Results
Mixing Container	138 L
Test Fluid	Water
Test Fluid Volume	103 L

Table XI   Control Function Test Results

Test Function	Expected Results	Acceptable (Yes/No)
Start Switch Operation	When the Start Switch is pressed, the mixer starts.	Yes
Stop Switch Operation	When the Stop Switch is pressed, the mixer stops.	Yes

6.3   Equipment Operation

6.3.1   Mixer Rotation Direction Test

Test Objective. The objective of this test is to verify that the mixer motor rotates in the proper direction. The mixer will be operated with the impeller being submerged in water.

Performed By:	Date:
Verified By:	Date:

℞ Equipment Qualification Protocol	Protocol No.: 4010
Title: (Any Mixer Co.) Model ME501 Emulsifying Mixer	Page: 12 of 21

Test Procedure

Materials and instruments required: mixing container, test fluid

- Fill the mixing container with water to its maximum working volume of 103 L and record the amount used in Table XII. When operating the mixer the head must be submerged in the water to prevent damage to the mixer.

    Test fluid volume calculation:

    Test fluid volume = 75% of 138 L = 103.5 L (rounded off to 103 L)

- Press the Start key and observe the direction of rotation of the mixer motor as viewed from the top of the mixer and record the results in Table XIII.

Table XII   Test Materials

Item	Results
Mixing Container	138 L
Test Fluid	Water
Test Fluid Volume	103 L

Table XIII   Mixer Motor Rotation Direction Test Results

Item	Expected Results	Results	Acceptable (Yes/No)
Mixer Motor Rotation Direction	Rotation should be clockwise as viewed from the top of the mixer.	Clockwise rotation was observed.	Yes
Performed By:			Date:
Verified By:			Date:

℞ Equipment Qualification Protocol	Protocol No.: 4010
Title: (Any Mixer Co.) Model ME501 Emulsifying Mixer	Page: 13 of 21

6.3.2 Mixer Speed Test

The speed test will not be performed during the OQ because the mixer cannot be operated without the impeller being submerged in water or other representative fluid or powder. This test is being performed in the PQ.

7.0 Performance Qualification (PQ)

Once it has been established that the equipment is properly installed and functioning within specified operating parameters, it must be shown that the mixer can be operated reliably under routine, minimum and maximum operating conditions.

7.1 Emulsifying Mixer Operation

Test Objective. The objective of this test is to document the performance of the mixer using water and a colored dye. Water will be used for maximum loading conditions. Also, the objective of this test is to verify that the mixer can move the fluid about the container (i.e., mixing). The speed of the mixer will be measured and recorded.

Test Procedure

Materials and instruments required: mixing container, test fluid, dye, tachometer

- Fill the mixing container with water to its maximum working volume of 103 L and record the amount used in Table XIV. When operating the mixer the head must be submerged in the water to prevent damage to the mixer.

Test Fluid Volume Calculation:

Test fluid volume = 75% of 138 L = 103.5 L (rounded off to 103 L)

Performed By:	Date:
Verified By:	Date:

℞ **Equipment Qualification Protocol**	Protocol No.: 4010
Title: (Any Mixer Co.) Model ME501 Emulsifying Mixer	Page: 14 of 21

- Turn the mixer on and observe the motion of the fluid and record the results in Table XV. The results of this test are qualitative only and are based on observation.

- Add FDC blue #1 dye to the water and observe the mixing action of the mixer and record the results in Table XV. Verify that the added dye is distributed uniformly throughout the container. Record the dye used in Table XIV.

- Measure the speed of the mixer with a calibrated tachometer. Verify that the measured speed is within $\pm 10\%$ of the fixed speed of 3480 rpm. Record the results in Table XVI and the instrument used to measure the speed in Table XVII.

Mixer Speed Calculation:

Mixer speed specification = 3480 rpm $\pm 10\%$
$\pm 10\%$ of 3480 = $\pm$ 348
3480 + 348 = 3828
3480 - 348 = 3132
The measured rpm of 3521 falls within $\pm 10\%$

Table **XIV**   Test Materials

Item	Results
Mixing Container	138 L
Test Fluid	Water
Dye	FDC Blue #1
Test Fluid Volume	103 L

Performed By:	Date:
Verified By:	Date:

℞ Equipment Qualification Protocol	Protocol No.: 4010
Title: (Any Mixer Co.) Model ME501 Emulsifying Mixer	Page: 15 of 21

Table XV Mixer Performance Test Results

Test Function	Expected Results	Results	Acceptable (Yes/No)
Fluid Mixing Capabilities	The mixer should move the fluid about the container.	Fluid motion and vortex action was observed. There was increased motion with increased speed.*	Yes
Fluid Mixing Capabilities	The added dye should be distributed uniformly throughout the container.	The dye was distributed uniformly throughout the container.*	Yes

* The results of this test are qualitative only, and are based on observation.

Table XVI Mixer Speed Test Results

Item	Specification rpm	Measured Speed rpm	Acceptable (Yes/No)
Mixer Speed	3480 ±10%	3521	Yes

Table XVII Instrument Used

Test Instrument	Identification Number	Calibration Due Date
Tachometer	64020	06/21/97

Performed By:	Date:
Verified By:	Date:

℞ **Equipment Qualification Protocol**	Protocol No.: 4010
Title: (Any Mixer Co.) Model ME501 Emulsifying Mixer	Page: 16 of 21

Attachment 1

Equipment Critical Instruments and
Test Equipment Calibration Certifications

R Equipment Qualification Protocol	Protocol No.: 4010
Title: (Any Mixer Co.) Model ME501 Emulsifying Mixer	Page: 17 of 21

Attachment 2

Calculation or Data Sheets

℞ Equipment Qualification Protocol	Protocol No.: 4010
Title: (Any Mixer Co.) Model ME501 Emulsifying Mixer	Page: 18 of 21

Attachment 3

Test Results

℞ Equipment Qualification Protocol	Protocol No.: 4010
Title: (Any Mixer Co.) Model ME501 Emulsifying Mixer	Page: 19 of 21

Attachment 4

Preventive Maintenance Schedule

R **Equipment Qualification Protocol**	Protocol No.: 4010	
Title: (Any Mixer Co.) Model ME501 Emulsifying Mixer		Page: 20 of 21

Attachment 5

Deficiencies

R Equipment Qualification Protocol	Protocol No.: 4010
Title: (Any Mixer Co.) Model ME501 Emulsifying Mixer	Page: 21 of 21

Attachment 6

Placebo Batch Records

Chapter 4

Protocol Writing through Approval

This chapter covers the next logical steps in the validation process: protocol writing, document review and approval, and project status. The methods that are described in this chapter apply to all of the validation department functions: cleaning, facilities, utilities, equipment, computer, software, and process.

PROTOCOL PREPARATION

After the equipment has been identified, priorities have been established, and writing projects have been assigned, it is time to start writing protocols. When I am starting a new equipment protocol writing project I go look at the equipment to get familiar with how it operates. Following are things to look for while viewing the equipment: the equipment number, which lets you know if you have the right piece of equipment; identification tags; facilities; utilities; control panel; motors; and how the equipment operates as a system. Then, back at my desk I make a copy of a protocol that is similar to the new one that I am getting ready to write. The first thing you have to know is what is the protocol number is going to be (see Chapter 8 under "Protocol Number Assignment Log" for the method used to assign the next protocol number.) Next, I enter the equipment's description. After determining the protocol number and equipment description, you have identified the protocol as your new writing project. Also, you need to obtain and read all of the following reference documentation to become familiar with the equipment.

Reference Documentation

The following reference documents are for a new piece of equipment or old equipment that has never been validated. Prior to writing any protocol, obtain copies of the following documentation and read, read, read. I will explain the use of each of the documentation items in the following list. This information will become part of the protocol documentation package that is archived in Document Control (see Chapter 8). This reference documentation establishes a baseline of documentation where protocol specifications reside for change control purposes (see Chapter 6).

Capitol appropriation request

Quote

Purchase requisition

Purchase order

Invoice

Packing slip

Vendor specification sheet

Vendor catalog

Equipment installation and operation manual

Equipment drawings

Spare parts list

Engineering standards

Standard operating procedures

Preventive maintenance schedule

Calibration certificates for equipment critical instruments

Calibration certificates for test instruments

- The capitol appropriation request, quote, purchase requisition, purchase order, invoice, and packing slip are used to establish a baseline of what was purchased. You do not need all of the above documents, but having them all would be helpful. The baseline will be used to compare what was purchased to what was received and installed, because if there are any differences they will have to be noted in the protocol.

- The vendor specification sheet, vendor catalog, equipment installation and operation manual, equipment drawings, spare parts list, and engineering standards are used to obtain equipment specifications that can be included in the protocol as challenge conditions during qualification testing. These specifications appear throughout the entire protocol.

- The equipment installation and operation manual and standard operating procedures are used to learn how to operate the equipment.

- The preventive maintenance schedule identifies which lubricants are used on the equipment. This schedule needs to be attached to the protocol for reference.

- The calibration certificates for equipment critical instruments and calibration certificates for test instruments need to be attached to the protocol for reference.

Next, I go through the protocol and start making changes based on the above information. Then I go look at the equipment again and watch how it operates—you see more things after reading the above information. The last thing I do is pretest the equipment. Pretesting the equipment eliminates most of the deviations, deficiencies, or addendums that occur from not knowing exactly how the equipment operates. You do not want any surprises during qualification testing because this can create down time and possible loss of product and shipments. You would like to have as clean a protocol as possible for FDA audits and for your own level of confidence.

Following are the methods that I use to obtain copies of the above reference documentation. Because some of the information has a longer lead time than others, I start sending out requests at the beginning of my writing project. I use memos as a method of retaining a record of what I requested and when. Then I keep copies of the memos in a folder to remind me of what I have sent out, and as they come in I close them out. Following are examples of ways to request invoices, purchase orders, calibration certifications, and preventive maintenance schedules.

MEMO

To: Finance

From: Validation

Date: September 19, 1998

Subject: REQUEST FOR COPIES OF EQUIPMENT INVOICES.

I need copies of the Invoice for the:

Bohle Tote Blender System PTM 200:   Asset No.: 5833

Bohle Blender LM 40:   Asset No.: 4933

I do not know the Purchase Order numbers. These pieces of equipment are in R&D.

MEMO

To: Purchasing

From: Validation

Date: June 29, 1998

Subject: REQUEST FOR COPIES OF PURCHASE ORDERS.

I need a copy of all of the Purchase Orders for the following pieces of equipment:

<u>PO Numbers</u>

Cremer Tablet & Capsule Counter:	164136
Lapel Capsealer:	212137
Kaps-All Capper:	510136
NJM Labeler:	003142
Omega Shrink Bundler:	003142
King Cottoner:	470136
Omega Bottle Unscrambler:	338138

Tablet Counter: Asset Number 1730 I don't know the Purchase Order number.

MEMO

To: Maintenance

From: Validation

Date: April 21, 1998

Subject: REQUEST FOR CALIBRATION CERTIFICATIONS.

I need copies of the calibration certifications for the MG Futura's
calibrated instruments.

Equipment Name	Calibration Number	Room Number	Department	Due Date
MG Futura	R&D-0731-GV-006 R&D-0731-MPR-009	147	R&D	4/17/98 10/17/97

MEMO

To: Maintenance

From: Validation

Date: June 12, 1998

Subject: REQUEST FOR PREVENTIVE MAINTENANCE SCHEDULE
          FOR ALL OF THE LINE 9 PIECES OF EQUIPMENT

These are new pieces of equipment, they might not even have a
preventive maintenance schedule.

Equipment	EQ. No.	Serial No.	Department
Cremer Tablet & Capsule Inserter	3141	334	Packaging line 9
Lepel Capsealer	3142	0-2080-35	Packaging line 9
Kaps-All Capper	3143	4048	Packaging line 9
NJM Labeler	3145	M97G112	Packaging line 9
Omega Shrink Bundler	3147	97J22253	Packaging line 9
King Cottoner	3148	2448/03	Packaging line 9
Kirby Tablet Counter	1730	LI1059	Packaging (Portable)

PROTOCOL WRITING TIPS

Following are the headings of all of the sections of the example protocol in Chapter 3 with some important writing tips.

Table of contents. A table of contents needs to be generated
if the protocol has more than 7 pages. The table of
contents shows the contents and attachments of the
protocol. The table of contents is generated automatically
from most software programs.

Objective. The objective of the equipment qualification is to establish documented evidence that the (equipment name) is acceptably installed per manufacturer recommendations, process requirements, and/or engineering standards. Acceptable installation includes suitable utility connections, components, and critical instruments in current calibration. Acceptable operation includes, as applicable, proper control and sequencing functions, recording and reporting functions, and safety and alarm features that meet process requirements and equipment specifications. Acceptable performance includes consistent operation within specified process parameters under simulated or actual production conditions.

Scope. The scope of the equipment qualification protocol includes the (equipment name) and its associated components. Installation qualification is limited to the system components and does not include installation of support utilities, other than the connections at the system boundary. Operational testing is limited to demonstrating equipment functionality. Product specific testing is outside the scope of this qualification protocol, other than where a product is used to demonstrate equipment functionality.

Equipment description. Include a brief narrative of the equipment and its intended use, appearance, capabilities, and operation method.

Installation Qualification

An IQ evaluation will establish confidence that the equipment is properly installed. The installation must meet the manufacturer's specified guidelines along with design changes at installation. Also, the supporting electrical utilities must meet all electrical codes. The information required for an IQ evaluation includes: equipment identification, required documentation, equipment utility requirements, major component specifications, component material, lubricants, and equipment safety features.

Equipment identification. This information is found on the nameplate (placard) attached to the equipment and in the equipment manufacturer's installation and operation manual.

Required documentation. Record the equipment manufacturer's operation and maintenance manual and drawings and your own standard operating procedures that cover the setup, operation, and cleaning of the equipment. The SOPs are listed separate from the other documentation because they have a release date. The dates on documentation furnished by the OEM are dates that they have established, and they are not necessarily the release date of that document. You need the release date for baselining and change control purposes, but the OEM does not usually provide it.

Equipment utility requirements. Record the volts, amps, compressed air pressure, water pressure, vacuum, and steam pressure. Record the instrument used to measure the volts, amps, compressed air pressure, water pressure, and steam pressure. Also, record the location of the power supply source.

Major component specification. Record the major components and verify that the components purchased were delivered and installed. This information is used for establishing a baseline and for change control purposes.

Component material. Record the material of each component that contacts the product.

Lubricants. Record the lubricant used to operate the equipment and indicate if the lubricant makes contact with the product.

Equipment safety features. List all safety features of the equipment.

Operational Qualification

An OQ evaluation should establish that the equipment can operate within specified tolerances and limits. The mechanical ranges of the equipment are being challenged along with the basic equipment operations. The equipment will be validated for its operating ability, not how well it performs an operation. The information required for the OQ evaluation includes: calibration of the instrument used to control the equipment, equipment control functions (switches and pushbuttons), and equipment operation (motor rotation direction and equipment speed).

Calibration requirements. Verify that all critical instruments on the equipment are logged into the calibration system, have calibration procedures in place, and are in calibration at the time of qualification testing. Record all of the necessary information for the calibrated instruments used to control the equipment. If there are no calibrated or non calibrated instruments on this equipment, so state in the protocol.

Equipment control functions.

Test objective. The objective of this test is to verify that the switches on the equipment operate per manufacturer specifications. You need to state clearly exactly what will be demonstrated and the expected results of the test. Objectives should be simple in nature, well thought out, and practical. Avoid terms that are ambiguous and open to interpretation.

Test procedure. The test needs to be outlined, thus allowing it to be executed in a practical manner. The instructions should be explicit to avoid misinterpretation and subsequent incorrect testing, but not so constricting as to preclude flexibility as operating conditions require. List all of the materials and instruments required to perform the qualification testing.

Test results. The raw data is recorded legibly. Errors and corrections in recording should be explained. If raw data is to be transcribed, attach the original data recorded to the protocol.

Equipment operation.

> **Test objective.** The objective of this test is to individually test each of the components and subcomponents of the system and verify that they operate per company requirements and manufacturer specifications.

Performance Qualification

Once it has been established that the equipment is properly installed and functioning within specified operating parameters, it must be shown that the equipment can be operated reliably under routine, minimum, and maximum operating conditions.

> **Test objective.** The objective of this test is to verify that the switches on the equipment operate per manufacturer specifications. You need to state clearly exactly what will be demonstrated and the expected results of the test. Objectives should be simple in nature, well thought out, and practical. Avoid terms that are ambiguous and open to interpretation.

> **Test procedure.** The test is outlined, allowing it to be executed in a practical manner. The instructions should be explicit to avoid misinterpretation and subsequent incorrect testing, but not so constricting as to preclude flexibility as field conditions require. List all of the materials and instruments required to perform the qualification testing.

> **Test results.** The raw data is recorded legibly. Errors and corrections in recording should be explained. If raw data is to be transcribed, attach the original data recorded to the protocol.

Protocol Attachments

The following documents must be attached to the protocol for reference.

> Equipment critical instrument and test equipment calibration certifications
>
> Calculation or data sheets
>
> Test results
>
> Preventive maintenance schedule
>
> Deficiencies
>
> Placebo batch records

DOCUMENT REVIEW AND APPROVAL

Now that the validation documentation has been written, it is time for review and approval by qualified individuals. First your document must be reviewed by your own department and then by outside departments. Review and approval will be required for each of the following documents: qualification and requalification protocols, final reports, conditional release forms, certification forms, validation baseline documents, deficiencies, and addendums. All of these documents will need to go through the Validation Change Control Board for review and approval (see Chapter 6). Following is an example of the flow of all validation documentation for review and approval.

✔ Department Review

First draft distributed for department review

Revise

Second draft distributed for department review

Revise

etc.

✔ Outside Department Review and Approval

The Validation Change Control Board becomes involved. The review board members review and approve all documents.

First draft distributed for outside department review

Revise

Second draft distributed for outside department review

Revise

etc.

Approval

Department Review

After you have finished writing your documents, you will need to distribute them for review and approval by your own department. Your documents will go through several iterations (as shown above) within your own department. Mark the first review copy "Draft 1"; this way department reviewers will know from the front of the document what part of the review cycle the document is in. The date is another method of determining which version you are sending out for review. When your documents come in from review you can tell at a glance the state of the document. When the document returns with reviewer comments marked in red, incorporate the changes and distribute Draft 2 and so forth until there are no more changes required. This allows you to have all of your ducks in a row before distributing your work to outside departments.

Now you are ready to distribute your department-reviewed documents to outside departments for review and approval. Do not sign the document at this time because this is just a draft copy, not the final.

Outside Department Review and Approval

Next, you will prepare a document review form (see the following paragraphs), attach a copy of the document to be reviewed, and then distribute the form simultaneously to all reviewers for comments or approval. There can only be one document per document review form. Give the reviewers a 1- or 2-week review time period (there is a place on the form for this). Tell them that they can return their comments to you or bring them to the next Validation Change Control Board meeting. You will go through the same iterations with the outside departments as you did with your own. Call the first distribution copy "Draft 1". When you get the document back marked-up in red, incorporate the changes and distribute Draft 2 and so forth until there are no more changes required.

The marked-up copies that you get back from each reviewer will be marked with either:

- Approved as is. The document is ready for use.

- Approved with conditions. You will need to show that the conditions have been met.

- Not approved. You will need to call a Validation Change Control Board meeting to resolve any issues. Also, when you get different department inputs that conflict with each other, you will need to call a Validation Change Control Board meeting to resolve those issues.

After all concerns have been addressed and changes incorporated, have your own department verify that you incorporated all of the changes correctly. Next, date and sign the document, then have your manager sign and date the document and bring it to the next Validation Change Control Board meeting. There, all board members will sign the document. After approval the document will be released into Document Control and then it is ready for use.

Document Review Form

With this form you will be answering the following questions:

- Who was the originator of the form and when did they check out the number?

- What is the document review form number?

- What is the document number and title?

- Which type of document is being reviewed?

- What was the reviewer's response?

- Who was the reviewer?

- Who were copies distributed to?

R̥	Document Review Form	
Originator: ❶	Date:	DRF No.: ❷

Document Number: ❸   Title:

Documentation Types: ❹

    ☐ Protocol ☐ Requal Protocol ☐ Final Report ☐ Conditional Release Form

    ☐ Certification Form ☐ Validation Baseline Document ☐ Deficiency

    ☐ Addendum

Reviewer Response: ❺

Select the appropriate option, then return your copy to validation. If no comments are received by (specified date) your concurrence will be assumed.

    ☐ Approved as is.

    ☐ Approved on condition that the attached comments are incorporated.

    ☐ Not approved, give reason.

Reviewer Signature: ❻	Date:

Distribution: ❼

Research & Development
Operations
Maintenance
Regulatory Compliance

Form Number: V002 (5/28/98)   Reference: SOP-VAL002

Document Review Form Preparation

Each circled number below corresponds to the circled number in the example document review form.

❶   Originator: Enter your name and date when you check out the number.

❷   DRF No.: Enter the next available document review form number (see Chapter 8 under "Document Review Form Number Assignment Log").

❸   Document Number: Enter the document number and title.

❹ Documentation Types: Mark the appropriate box for the document that needs to be reviewed and approved.

❺ Reviewer Response: The Reviewer marks the appropriate response after your review.

❻ Reviewer Signature: The reviewer signs and dates when your review is complete.

❼ Distribution: List who copies were distributed to. This is your standard distribution for all documents.

℞	**Document Review Form**	
Originator:	Date:	DRF No.: 001

Document Number: FR001

Title: (Any Mixer Co.) Model ME501 Emulsifying Mixer

Documentation Types:

☐ Protocol   ☐ Requal Protocol   ☒ Final Report   ☐ Conditional Release Form

☐ Certification Form   ☐ Validation Baseline Document   ☐ Deficiency

☐ Addendum

Reviewer Response:

Select the appropriate option, then return your copy to validation. If no comments are received by (10/20/98) your concurrence will be assumed.

☒ Approved as is.

☐ Approved on condition that the attached comments are incorporated.

☐ Not approved, give reason.

Reviewer Signature:	Date:

Distribution:

   Research & Development
   Operations
   Maintenance
   Regulatory Compliance

Form Number: V002 (5/28/98)   Reference: SOP-VAL002

Document Review Form Number Assignment

The numbering systems in this part of the book are for manual paperbased documentation systems. In the paperbased system you will need logbooks to record your documentation numbers. Using logbooks allows you to see what the next available number is when you need to assign a new number. There needs to be a logbook in Document Control where document review form numbers are assigned (see Chapter 8 under "Document Review Form Number Assignment Log").

PROJECT STATUS LIST

Now that writing projects have started and the protocols are out for review and approval you will need a method of keeping track of where the protocols are and what their status is at all times. A project status list can be used to keep track of all of your projects on a daily basis. The list can be developed and updated in a spreadsheet. Following is a simple method for keeping track of your protocol writing projects. With this list you will be answering the following questions:

- What is the protocol number?
- What was the start date?
- Which protocols need to be written?
- Are the protocols being written?
- Are the protocols out for review?
- Are changes being incorporated?
- Are protocols ready for qualification testing?
- Is qualification testing complete?
- Is the final report written?
- What is the complete date?

℞	**Project Status List**			
Protocol Number →	❶			
Events ↓ ❷				
Need to Write				
Start Writing				
Out for Review				
Incorporating Changes				
Out for Review				
Qual or Requal Testing				
Writing Final Report				
Out For Review				
Incorporating Changes				
Out for Review				
Complete Date				
etc.				

Project Status List Preparation

Each circled number below corresponds to the circled number on the example project status list.

❶   Protocol Number: Enter the protocol numbers to the right.

❷   Events: Enter all of the dates for each of the events below the applicable protocol.

℞	Project Status List			
Protocol Number →	2007	3089 A	4010 D	5023
Events ↓				
Need to Write	01/10/98	01/10/98	01/10/98	01/10/98
Start Writing	02/28/98	02/27/98	02/26/98	03/29/98
Out for Review		02/28/98	03/18/98	05/06/98
Incorporating Changes		03/07/98	03/28/98	
Out for Review		03/29/98	03/29/98	
Qual or Requal Testing		04/30/98	04/30/98	
Writing Final Report			04/31/98	
Out For Review			05/04/98	
Incorporating Changes			05/06/98	
Out for Review			05/07/98	
Complete Date			06/10/98	
etc.				

Chapter 5

Qualification Testing through Certification

This chapter covers the next logical steps in the validation process: qualification testing, final reports, conditional release, and system certification. Equipment qualification testing is covered in great detail in a companion volume published by Interpharm Press, *Pharmaceutical Equipment Validation: The Ultimate Qualification Guidebook.*

QUALIFICATION TESTING

It is important that you prepare written qualification protocols that specify the tests to be conducted and the data to be collected. The reason for collecting test data must be clearly understood, and your observations must be documented. The test data must reflect reality and be recorded accurately. The protocol should specify a sufficient number of tests to show repeatability and provide an accurate assessment of the variability of consecutive runs. The test conditions for these runs should impose upper and lower control limits. A thorough analysis will ensure that the control limits for the equipment are appropriate and that it will not fail if operated within those limits. Testing all function at the extremes of operation and showing those limits to be acceptable will provide assurance that the intermediate levels are acceptable. You are validating the equipment for its mechanical parameters, not how well it processes something. For example, a mixer will be validated for minimum and maximum speeds, loading, etc., not how well it mixes powders. How well it mixes powders pertains to process validation, not equipment validation.

Qualification testing requires knowledge of how to measure volts, amps, motor speeds, revolutions per minute, time, temperature, air pressure, vacuum, water pressure, steam pressure, flow rates, mechanical dimensions, volumes, etc. You will also be calculating weights, volumes, and averages; establishing tolerances; and reading and interpreting gauges installed on the equipment and the test instruments used to take measurements. You will need to know what type of control system is involved in the operation of the equipment, such as automatic, semi-automatic, or manual. An automatic system is controlled by a microprocessor, PLC, or PC while a manual system is regulated by adjustments made by the operator.

What Needs to Be Tested?

Everything on a piece of equipment needs to be validated in one way or another; the question is how much and to what detail. This one is easy—if it moves, test it. Validate the equipment that makes contact with the product first, then work your way out from there. Definition of what needs to be validated:

Utensil: A device that has no control specifications and takes no measurements. An example of this would be a device that would replace what an operator would do by hand (i.e., stir plates, stir rods, and spatulas). Utensils do not need to be validated. Glassware that is used to measure a volume is certified by the vendor.

Instrument: A device that takes a physical measurement and displays a value, but has no control or analytical function (i.e., stopwatches, timers, and thermometers). Instruments do not need to be validated, but do require initial and ongoing calibration programs.

Equipment: A device or collection of components that perform a process to produce a result, such as producing an environment or performing an action on something. Equipment needs to be validated.

You can use the following methods to obtain a list of components that need to be tested.

- Observe the equipment in operation

- Obtain major components from the equipment manufacturer's installation and operation manual and spare parts list

What Level of Testing Is Required?

Several attempts have been made throughout the industry to establish a test standard for equipment challenge conditions. Listed below are the test standards that I have found to date. Before you decide which test condition to use, find out what the normal operating conditions are for the piece of equipment to be tested from the equipment operator. Then pick a challenge condition from the following list. What you are trying to gain by testing is a level of confidence that the equipment is operating under a state of control.

- Minimum/maximum operating ranges
  This applies to utilities, motor speeds, time, temperature, air pressure, vacuum, water pressure, steam pressure, flow rates, weights, volumes, etc.

- Minimum/maximum load evaluations
  This applies to mixers, blenders, etc. Each company needs to have standards stating that if the equipment is operated above or below these limits you will not have good results. Your testing should go outside these limits.

- Most appropriate challenge condition

I do not like this test because the word "appropriate" leaves this open for interpretation.

- Effective ranges of critical parameters
The problem with this test is the word "critical". If you ask several people which components on a piece of equipment are the most critical, you will get several different answers.

- Proven acceptable range (PAR) and range of experience
These tests do not apply to new equipment. The only problem with these is that the ranges are not necessarily the minimum and maximum ranges.

- Intended range of use
I use this test a lot. The only problem with it is that the ranges are not necessarily the minimum and maximum ranges.

- Worst Case
This is the test you hear about most often. It is similar to the minimum/maximum load evaluations and minimum/maximum ranges.

- Edge of failure
Of course, this does not apply to equipment because you would have to make something fail to obtain the edge failure, although it could apply to the product. For example, the point where a tablet is destroyed is just past the edge of failure. Therefore, you could back off that number and call it the tablets edge of failure.

How Much Testing Is Enough?

Question: What is an acceptable number of times a process step needs to be repeated successfully to say an operation is validated: three (so that you can have an average) 10, 100, or 1000?

Answer: The number of repetitions of a process step during qualification should be based on statistical significance. There is a conventional wisdom about validation that once is chance, twice is nice, and three times is validation. Because of these reasons, validation is often performed over three trials. Three should be considered a minimum. Sometimes, however, the experimental design may dictate that a higher level of confidence is required to prove the process. The number of units or duration of trials used in validation is also intended to represent a typical production lot size or production duration. The key words from the above are "confidence level" and "statistical significance". You can look them up in (*Juran's Quality Control Handbook* (see Appendix J for more information). Statistical process control is beyond the scope of this book.

FINAL REPORT

This section covers the final report format and its use. The following example is for an equipment qualification. The final report is written after all of the qualification and requalification testing is complete. It is written by a validation specialist and

Figure 5.1   **Final Report Contents**

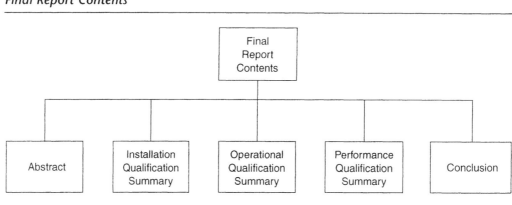

approved by the validation manager, Research and Development, Operations, Maintenance, and Regulatory Compliance. The final report is made up of the following elements: abstract, IQ, OQ, PQ, conclusion (Fig. 5.1).

The final report should be in narrative form and written in simple language that describes in general terms the significant aspects of the entire qualification package. The final report is designed to condense the data generated during the execution of qualification testing. Statements summarizing the important points of the qualification testing should be included. The final report will contain the results of the overall testing and conclude the results of the data.

All deviations should be detailed and cross referenced to the protocol along with any deficiencies or addendums and the actions taken to correct and/or respond to them. Upon approval, the final report will become part of the qualification and requal protocol package and placed in Document Control (see Chapter 8 under "Protocol Package Contents Sheet").

This section will show you how to develop a complete final report. The method of development applies the same to all validation department functions. What you need to do is capture the most pertinent information that identifies which qualification you are reporting on, which system is being validated, and who prepared and approved the final report. Following is an example of the first page of a final report. The information for the header comes from the qualification protocol itself. Note that the same people who sign a protocol need to sign the final report in the footer. I have made cross references in the final report to an addendum, a deficiency, and a deviation (see Chapter 6).

Final Report Form

With the final report you will be answering the following questions:

- What is the protocol number and title?
- What is the final report number?
- Who is the equipment manufacturer?
- What is the model number and the serial number?

- What is the equipment number?
- What was the location of the equipment at the time of testing?
- Who prepared the final report?
- Who reviewed and approved the final report?
- Which equipment was validated?
- Was the qualification testing successful?

R̽	Final Report		
Protocol No.:　❶ Title:		FR No.:　❷	
Manufacturer:　　　　❸		Page:　❹	
Model Number:　❺	Serial Number:　❻		
Equipment Number:　❼	Location:　❽		
Cover Page			
❾　　　　Prepared By:			
Validation:			Date:
❿　　　　Approved By:			
Validation Manager:			Date:
Research & Development:			Date:
Operations:			Date:
Maintenance:			Date:
Regulatory Compliance:			Date:

Final Report – Page 1 Preparation

Each circled number below corresponds to the circled number on page 1 of the example final report.

❶   Protocol No.: Enter the protocol number and title (see Chapter 2 under "Protocol Numbering System" and "Protocol Title").

Example: 4010 (Any Mixer Co.) Model ME501 Emulsifying Mixer

❷   FR No.: Enter the next available final report number (see Chapter 8 under "Final Report Number Assignment Log").

Example: FR001

❸   Manufacturer: Enter the name of the manufacturer.

❹   Page: Enter the page number.

Example: Page 1 of 4
This method is best for change control purposes because you will have to account for every page of the final report.

❺   Model Number: Enter the model number.

❻   Serial Number: Enter the serial number.

❼   Equipment Number: Enter the equipment number (see Chapter 2 under "Equipment Numbering System").

Example: Minor Equipment Number: 00
Major Equipment Number: 000

❽   Location: Enter the location of the equipment when it was tested, even if it is portable.

❾   Prepared By: Enter your name and date when the final report is complete.

❿   Approved By: Each reviewer enter your name and date when your review and approval is complete.

Final Report – Page 2

Following is an example of the second page of a final report. You do not need to repeat the complete page 1 header on the subsequent pages. The information for the header comes from page 1 of the final report.

Final Report – Page 2 Preparation

Each circled number below corresponds to the circled number on page 2 of the sample final report.

❶   Protocol No.: Enter the protocol number (same as page 1).

❷   FR No.: Enter the final report number (same as page 1).

❸   Protocol Title: Enter the protocol title (same as page 1).

R̝	Final Report		
Protocol No.: ❶		FR No.: ❷	
Protocol Title: ❸		Page No.: ❹	

Subsequent Pages

❹   Page No.: Enter the page number.

Example: Page 2 of 4

This method is best for change control purposes because you will have to account for every page of the final report.

Completed Final Report

I have included an actual equipment final report template that is filled in, thus showing you how to develop a final report by example. Each of the aforementioned final report elements is covered in the template.

℞	Final Report		
Protocol No.: 4056 Title: (Any Mixer Co.) Model GM200 Capsule Filler		FR No.: 001	
Manufacturer: Any Encapsulator Co.		Page: 1 of 2	
Model Number: GM200		Serial Number: Y67291	
Equipment Number: 371		Location: Room 539	

<table>
<tr><td colspan="3">

Abstract

The encapsulator is a new piece of equipment that is made up of several major components. It is controlled by a programmable logic controller (PLC). On the powder dosing unit the powder chamber, compression and layer values are modified by drives that are integrated in the machine logic and controlled by the PLC. The pellet dosing unit is entirely integrated in the machine logic and handled by the PLC.

The software program was evaluated against the functional requirements and the intended use of the equipment. The EEPROM was removed from the machine by the vendor so they could make changes at their home office. The program that was on the EEPROM was loaded into the RAM of the PLC so that the machine could be operated. The new software upgrade was received and installed. See Addendum A023, against protocol 4056.

</td></tr>
<tr><td colspan="3" align="center">**Prepared By:**</td></tr>
<tr><td colspan="2">Validation:</td><td>Date:</td></tr>
<tr><td colspan="3" align="center">**Approved By:**</td></tr>
<tr><td colspan="2">Validation Manager:</td><td>Date:</td></tr>
<tr><td colspan="2">Research & Development:</td><td>Date:</td></tr>
<tr><td colspan="2">Operations:</td><td>Date:</td></tr>
<tr><td colspan="2">Maintenance:</td><td>Date:</td></tr>
<tr><td colspan="2">Regulatory Compliance:</td><td>Date:</td></tr>
</table>

R̥	Final Report	
Protocol No.: 4056		FR No.: 001
Protocol Title: (Any Encapsulator Co.) Model GM200 Capsule Filler		Page: 2 of 2

Installation Qualification

The unit was installed properly and all components were present. All applicable procedures were in place. The utilities supplied to the unit were inspected and found to be acceptable for proper operation of the unit.

Operational Qualification

All control and operational test function results were acceptable per the protocol test requirements. All alarms and safety devices functioned acceptably per the protocol test requirements except for the door interlocks that did not operate properly. See attached deficiency DF075 against protocol 4056.

Performance Qualification

All performance testing was acceptable per the protocol test requirements. The following item was a deviation from the original qualification protocol.

Dev. No.	Deviation	Protocol Page(s)
1	The original speed was measured with a hand held tachometer. This information was lined out and initialed and dated and a new measurement was taken with a calibrated remote speed controller that was specifically manufactured for this equipment.	21

Conclusion

The capsule filler has been tested and verified to operate properly according to manufacturer and process specifications. All corrections were noted in the protocol and a deficiency and an addendum were required.

Figure 5.2   **System Release Methods**

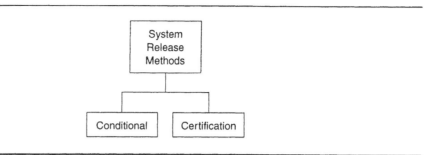

Final Report Number Assignment

The numbering systems in this part of the book are for manual paperbased documentation systems. In the paperbased system you will need logbooks to record your documentation numbers. Using logbooks allows you to see what the next available number is when you need to assign a new number. There needs to be a logbook in Document Control where document review form numbers are assigned (see Chapter 8 under "Final Report Number Assignment Log").

CONDITIONAL RELEASE AND SYSTEM CERTIFICATION

This section covers the conditional release and certification of cleaning, facilities, utilities, equipment, computer, software, and process validations. The forms can be initiated by any member of the validation department. The validation department releases facilities, equipment, and computer systems for operational use upon completion of qualification testing. The release can occur in one of two methods: Conditional or Certification (Fig. 5.2).

Conditional Release

A system cannot be used until it has been validated. The system can be conditionally released after the qualification or requalification testing is complete and verified, and prior to the completion of the final report. Usually the system owner is waiting to use the system, therefore this method can be used to expedite the validation process by allowing the system owner to use the system prior to completion of all of the documentation.

Conditional Release Form

With this form you will be answering the following questions:

- What is the protocol number and title?
- What is the conditional release form number?
- Who is the manufacturer?
- What is the model number?
- What is the serial number?
- What is the equipment number (if applicable)?

- What is the equipment number (if applicable)?
- What is the location of the equipment (if applicable)?
- Which department owns the system?
- What date was the system conditionally released?
- Who originated the conditional release form?
- Who reviewed and approved the conditional release?

R̥	**Conditional Release Form**	
Protocol Number: ❶ Title:		CRF No.: ❷
Manufacturer: ❸		
Model Number: ❹	Serial Number: ❺	
Equipment Number: ❻	Location: ❼	

❽

Statement

All of the qualification testing and verification is complete, therefore, the (system name) is released for use by (Department Name).

Conditional Release Date: (03/15/99)

Originator: ❾	Date:
Approved By: Validation Manager: ❿	Date:

Form Number: V003 (5/28/98)   Reference: SOP-VAL003

Conditional Release Form Preparation

Each circled number below corresponds to the circled number in the sample conditional release form.

❶ Protocol Number: Enter the protocol number and title (see Chapter 2 under "Protocol Numbering System" and "Protocol Title").

Example: 4010 (Any Mixer Co.) Model ME501 Emulsifying Mixer

❷ CRF No.: Enter the next available conditional release form number (see Chapter 8 under "Conditional Release Form Number Assignment Log").

Example: CRF001

❸ Manufacturer: Enter the name of the manufacturer.

❹ Model Number: Enter the model number.

❺ Serial Number: Enter the serial number.

❻ Equipment Number: Enter the equipment number (see Chapter 2 under "Equipment Numbering System").

Example: Minor Equipment Number: 00
Major Equipment Number: 000

❼ Location: Enter the location of the equipment when it was tested, even if it is portable.

❽ Statement: Enter the system name, equipment owner's department, and the conditional release date.

❾ Originator: Enter your name and the date.

❿ Approved By: The validation manager will sign and date the form when the qualification testing is complete and verified, prior to the completion of the final report.

Completed Conditional Release Form

I have included an actual conditional release form template that is filled in, thus showing you how to develop a conditional release form by example. Each of the aforementioned conditional release elements is covered in the template.

Conditional Release Form Number Assignment

There needs to be a logbook in Document Control where conditional release form numbers are assigned (see Chapter 8 under "Conditional Release Form Number Assignment Log").

System Certification

A system cannot be used until it has been certified. The system can be certified after the qualification or requalification testing is complete and verified, and after the final report is complete. Following is an example of a certification form. The

R̶	**Conditional Release Form**	
Protocol No.: 4010 Title: (Any Mixer Co.) Model ME501 Emulsifying Mixer		CRF No.: 001
Manufacturer: Any Mixer Co.		
Model Number: MC501	Serial Number: 55356 B	
Equipment Number: 205	Location: Room 802 (This equipment is portable.)	

Statement

All of the qualification testing and verification is complete, therefore, the **Model ME501 Emulsifying Mixer** is released for use by Operations.

Conditional Release Date: (06/10/98)

Originator:	Date:
Approved By:	
Validation Manager:	Date:

Form Number: V003 (5/28/98)   Reference: SOP-VAL003

information for the certification comes from the qualification or requal protocol. With this form you will be answering the following questions:

- What is the protocol number and title?

- What is the certification form number?

- Who is the manufacturer?

- What is the model number?

- What is the serial number?

- What is the equipment number (if applicable)?

- What is the location of the equipment (if applicable)?

- Which system is being certified?

- Who originated the certification form?

- Who reviewed and approved the certification?

Ŗ	**Certification Form**	
Protocol No.: ❶ Title:		CF No.: ❷
Manufacturer: ❸		
Model Number: ❹	Serial Number: ❺	
Equipment Number: ❻	Location: ❼	

❽

Statement

Based upon the acceptable results of the qualification testing and any applicable follow-up actions, this (system name) has been found to meet all validation requirements defined herein.

Certification Date: (06/10/98)

Originator: ❾	Date:
Approved By: Manager of Validation: ❿	Date:

Form Number: V004 (5/28/98)   Reference: SOP-VAL004

Certification Form Preparation

Each circled number below corresponds to the circled number in the sample certification form.

❶ Protocol No.: Enter the protocol number and title (see Chapter 2 under "Protocol Numbering System" and "Protocol Title").

Example: 4010 (Any Mixer Co.) Model ME501 Emulsifying Mixer

❷ CF No.: Enter the next available certification form number (see Chapter 8 under "Certification Form Number Assignment Log").

Example: CF001

❸ Manufacturer: Enter the name of the manufacturer.

❹ Model Number: Enter the model number.

❺ Serial Number: Enter the serial number.

❻ Equipment Number: Enter the equipment number (see Chapter 2 under "Equipment Numbering System").

Example: Minor Equipment Number: 00
Major Equipment Number: 000

❼ Location: Enter the location of the equipment when it was tested, even if it is portable.

❽ Statement: Enter the system name and the certification date.

❾ Originator: Enter your name and date.

❿ Approved By: The validation manager will sign and date the form when the qualification testing and final report are complete and approved and all deviations and deficiencies have been resolved.

Completed Certification Form

I have included an actual certification template that is filled in, thus showing you how to develop a certification form by example. Each of the aforementioned certification elements is covered in this template.

Certification Form Number Assignment

There needs to be a logbook in Document Control where certification form numbers are assigned (see Chapter 8 under "Certification Form Number Assignment Log").

VALIDATION RELEASE TAG

A validation release tag will be affixed to the system upon the release of that system for use, either conditional or certified (see Fig. 5.3). The tag indicates that the system has been initially qualified or requalified and released by validation. This

℞	Certification Form	
Protocol No.: 4010 Title: (Any Mixer Co.) Model ME501 Emulsifying Mixer		CF No.: CF001
Manufacturer: Any Mixer Co.		
Model Number: MC501	Serial Number: 55356 B	
Equipment Number: 2052	Location: Room 802 (This equipment is portable.)	

Statement

Based upon the acceptable results of the qualification testing and any applicable follow-up actions, this **Model ME501 Emulsifying Mixer** has been found to meet all validation requirements defined herein.

Certification Date: (06/10/98)

Originator:	Date:
Approved By: Manager of Validation:	Date:

Form Number: V004 (5/28/98)   Reference: SOP-VAL004

Figure 5.3   *Validation Release Tag*

Validation Release
☐ Conditional   ☐ Certified
Date:

signifies that the validation documentation has been generated, reviewed, approved, and tested and that the system is in the validation document control system, which includes change control.

Chapter 6

Change Control

This Chapter covers the next logical steps in the validation process: baseline management and change control. Change control is comprised of the Validation Change Control Board, validation change request form, deviations, deficiency form, and addendums. The methods that are described in this chapter apply to all of the validation department functions: cleaning, facilities, utilities, equipment, computer, software, and process.

BASELINE MANAGEMENT

Baseline management comes into play after documents are completed and placed in Document Control. The documents become a part of a baseline freeze, which means that nothing can be changed without going through the Validation Change Control System. Fig. 6.1 shows which documents need to be baselined. Baseline freezes will assure that each archived document is under a state of control at all times. Each separate protocol will have its own validation baseline document.

Protocol packages need to have a validation baseline document created because they are comprised of documents from several sources inside and outside of the company (see the following list). A baseline document establishes a record of the release and/or revision dates of the protocol and its reference documents. Plans, policies, SOPs, and engineering studies are stand alone documents and do not need a validation baseline document, but they will be reviewed and approved by the Validation Change Control Board.

Figure 6.1   **Validation Documentation**

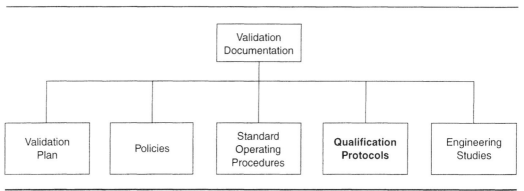

Document Sources

Validation

Equipment user

Finance

Purchasing

Maintenance

Calibration

Original equipment manufacturer

Vendors

Validation Baseline Document

This section will show you how to develop a complete validation baseline document; the method of development applies to all validation department functions. You need to capture the most pertinent information that identifies which qualification this is, which equipment is being validated (if applicable), and who prepared and approved the validation baseline document. With the validation baseline document you will be answering the following questions:

- What is the protocol number and title?

- What is the validation baseline document number?

- Who is the equipment manufacturer?

- What is the model number and the serial number?

- What is the equipment number?

- What was the location of the equipment at the time of testing?

- Who prepared the validation baseline document?

- Who reviewed and approved the validation baseline document?

- Which equipment is being validated?

- Which system was baselined?

℞	**Validation Baseline Document**		
Protocol Number: ❶ Title:		VBD No.: ❷	
Manufacturer: ❸		Page: ❹	
Model Number: ❺	Serial Number: ❻		
Equipment Number: ❼	Location: ❽		

Cover Page

⑨ Prepared By:		
Validation:		Date:
⑩ Approved By:		
Validation Manager:		Date:
Research & Development:		Date:
Operations:		Date:
Maintenance:		Date:
Regulatory Compliance:		Date:

Form Number: V005 (5/28/98)   Page 1 of 2   Reference: SOP-VAL005

Validation Baseline Document–Page 1 Preparation

Each circled number below corresponds to the circled number in the sample validation baseline document.

❶   Protocol Number: Enter the protocol number and title (see Chapter 2 under "Protocol Numbering System" and "Title").

Example: 4010 (Any Mixer Co.) Model ME501 Emulsifying Mixer

❷   VBD No.: Enter the next available validation baseline document number (see Chapter 8 under "Validation Baseline Document Number Assignment Log").

Example: VBD001

❸   Manufacturer: Enter the name of the manufacturer.

❹   Page: Enter the page number.

Example: Page 1 of 9

This method is best for change control purposes because you will need to account for every page of the validation baseline document.

❺   Model Number: Enter the model number.

❻   Serial Number: Enter the serial number.

❼   Equipment Number: Enter the equipment number (see Chapter 2 under "Equipment Numbering System").

Example: Minor Equipment Number: 00
        Major Equipment Number: 000

❽   Location: Enter the location of the equipment when it was tested, even if it is portable.

❾   Prepared By: Enter your name and date when the validation baseline document is complete.

❿   Approved By: Each reviewer enter your name and date when your review and approval is complete.

Validation Baseline Document – Page 2

Following is an example of the second page of a validation baseline document. You do not need to repeat the entire header on subsequent pages; you only need the information that identifies the equipment that is being validated, the protocol number, and the page number.

Validation Baseline Document – Page 2 Preparation

Each circled number below corresponds to the circled number on the subsequent pages of the sample validation baseline document.

❶   Protocol Number: Enter the protocol number and title (same as page 1).

❷   VBD No.: Enter the validation baseline document number (same as page 1).

❸   Page: Enter the page number.

Example: Page 2 of 9

This method is best for change control purposes because you will need to account for every page of the validation baseline document.

❹   Document Number: Enter the document number starting with protocol numbers.

R̥	Validation Baseline Document		
Protocol Number: **❶**		VBD No.: **❷**	
Title:		Page: **❸**	
Document Number	Description		Release Date
❹	**❺**		**⑥**

Form Number: V005 (5/28/98)   Page 2 of 2   Reference: SOP-VAL005

❺   Description: Enter the document's description.

⑥   Release Date: Enter the release or revision date of the document.

VALIDATION BASELINE DOCUMENT NUMBER ASSIGNMENT

The numbering systems in this part of the book are for manual paperbased documentation systems. In the paperbased system you will need logbooks to record your documentation numbers. Using logbooks allows you to see what the next available

℞	**Validation Baseline Document**	
Protocol No.: 4010 Title: (Any Mixer Co.) Model ME501 Emulsifying Mixer		VBD No.: 001
Manufacturer: Any Mixer Co.		Page: 1 of 2
Model Number: MC501	Serial Number: 55356 B	
Equipment Number: 2052	Location: Room 802 (This equipment is portable.)	

Prepared By:	
Validation:	Date:
Approved By:	
Validation Manager:	Date:
Research & Development:	Date:
Operations:	Date:
Maintenance:	Date:
Regulatory Compliance:	Date:

Form Number: V005 (5/28/98)   Page 1 of 2   Reference: SOP-VAL005

number is when you need to assign a new number. There needs to be a logbook in Document Control where validation baseline document numbers are assigned (see Chapter 8 under "Validation Baseline Document Number Assignment Log").

CHANGE CONTROL SYSTEM

Once a system has been considered validated, the FDA requires that the system remains unchanged. Change control keeps a record of all changes to a system

℞	Validation Baseline Document		
Protocol No.: 4010		VBD No.: 001	
Title: (Any Mixer Co.) Model ME501 Emulsifying Mixer		Page: 2 of 2	
Document Number	Description	Release Date	
CF001	Certification, Equipment	05/07/98	
FR001	Final Report	05/07/98	
DF001	Deficiency	02/17/98	
A001	Addendum	03/19/98	
67792	Capitol Appropriations Request	06/10/95	
Q2542	Quote	06/15/98	
PR02576	Purchase Requisition	07/09/95	
PO12157	Purchase Order	07/24/95	
8110	Invoice	11/21/95	
77512	Packing Slip	12/02/95	
3.67.4	Vendor Spec Sheet	03/16/92	
4.21	Vendor Catalog: Model ME501 Emulsifying Mixer	03/16/97	
M37219	Manual: Installation and Operation of Model ME501	05/16/97	
D-1346	Drawing: Standard Production Mixer Emulsifier	05/26/97	
OPS026	SOPs: Model ME501 Emulsifying Mixer Set-Up, Operation and Cleaning	11/02/97	
ES116	Engineering Standard: High Shear Granulator Mixers	12/19/97	
00651	Preventive Maintenance Schedule: Monthly and 6 months	04/26/98	
012-ETM	Calibration Certificates- Equipment Critical Instruments	06/19/98	
None	Calibration Certificates-Test Instruments		
SPL4567	Spare Parts List	05/16/95	

Form Number: V005 (5/28/98)   Page 2 of 2   Reference: SOP-VAL005

that provides assurance that a state of control exists. A formal system that regulates and documents any requested and implemented changes needs to be in place. Even though a single change might not affect a system, several changes over a period of time could have an adverse effect. A cross reference list that keeps track of all of the changes against each baselined system is necessary. This list can be developed and changed using spreadsheet software. The cross reference list will cross reference the validation change request forms, deficiencies, and addendums to the baselined systems.

Figure 6.2   *Change Control System*

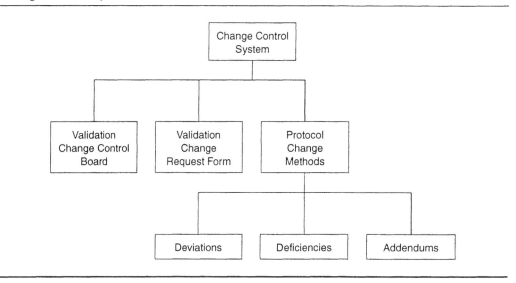

Reasons for Changes

Following are some of the reasons for making changes to baselined validation protocols.

New equipment

Equipment has been relocated

Equipment has been modified

Major mechanical equipment has been replaced

Critical items have been replaced or repaired

Cleaning process changed

Product changed

Process changed

System upgrades have been added

Computer systems have been replaced

Additions to the functionality of the system have been made

Time

A lot of changes have been made

Regulatory requirements have changed

Records were lost

This section covers all of the change control methods used to keep the validation system and documentation within a validated state of control (see Fig. 6.2). Changing qualification and requalification protocols, establishing a validation change control board, preparing a validation change request form, documenting deviations, preparing a deficiency form, and preparing addendums are discussed. The methods described in this section apply to all of the validation department functions: cleaning, facilities, utilities, equipment, computer, software, and process.

Validation Documentation

Now that a baseline of validation documentation has been established, it's time to start managing changes to that system. A change control method that will handle changes to any of the following validation documents must be in place. All of the documents listed below will be reviewed and approved by the validation change control board.

> Certifications
>
> Final reports
>
> Protocols
>
> Requal protocols
>
> Deficiencies
>
> Addendums
>
> Engineering studies
>
> Validation plans
>
> Policies
>
> SOPs

Validation Change Control Board

Establish a change control board with representation from key personnel (Fig. 6.3). Rigorous change control and detailed documentation is absolutely necessary to make sure previous validation efforts have not been lost. Change control starts when validation documentation has been approved and released into Document Control. From this time on every change to any of the documents must go through the Validation Change Control Board.

Validation Change Request Form

The change control process starts with a request to make a change to a baselined system. Anyone can request a change by preparing the validation change request form. This section will show you how to complete a validation change request form. The method of preparation applies the same for all validation department functions. Validation change requests will be reviewed and approved by the Validation Change Control Board. You need to capture the most pertinent information that identifies what qualification this is, which equipment is being validated (if any), and who prepared and approved the validation change request form. With the validation change request form you will be answering the following questions:

- Who was the originator of the form and when was it originated?

- What is the validation change request form number?

Figure 6.3   *Validation Change Control Board*

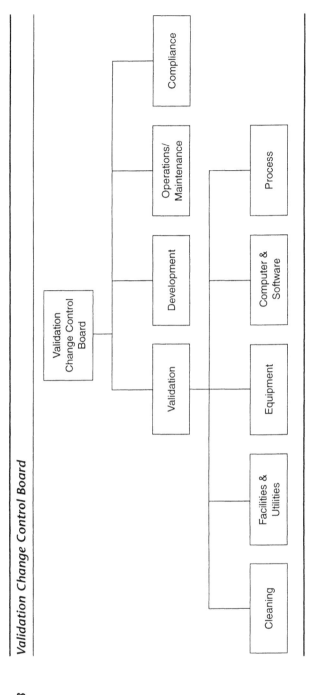

℞	Validation Change Request Form		
Originator: ❶ Date:		VCRF No.: ❷	

Validation Baseline Affected: ❸	Priority: ❹
☐ Cleaning ☐ Facility ☐ Utility ☐ Equipment ☐ Computer ☐ Software ☐ Process ☐ Requal	☐ Routine ☐ Urgent

Documents Affected:		
Document Number	Revision	Title
❺	❻	❼

Reason and Description of Change or (See marked-up documents):

❽

Corrective Action: ⑨

⑩ Approved By:		
Validation Manager:	Date:
Research & Development:	Date:
Operations:	Date:
Maintenance:	Date:
Regulatory Compliance:	Date:

Form Number: V006 (5/28/98)   Reference: SOP-VAL006

- Which validation baseline is affected by this change?

- What is the priority of the change request?

- Which documents are affected by the change?

- What is the reason for and description of the change?

- What corrective action is required?

- Who reviewed and approved the validation change request form?

Validation Change Request Form Preparation

Each circled number below corresponds to the circled number in the sample validation change request form format.

❶   Originator: Enter your name and date when validation change request form is complete.

❷   VCRF No.: Enter the next available validation change request form number (see Chapter 8 under "Validation Change Request Form Number Assignment Log").

Example: VCRF001

❸   Validation Baseline Affected: Mark the appropriate box based on which validation function(s) is (are) affected.

❹   Priority: Mark the appropriate box depending on the priority of the change.

❺   Document Number: Enter the numbers of all of the documents that are affected by this change.

❻   Revision: Enter the revision or the date of the affected document(s).

❼   Title: Enter the title of the affected document(s).

❽   Reason and Description of Change: Enter the reason and description of the change or attach marked-up documents. Tip: This always seems to be a hard one for everybody. Think of it as what would happen if you did not make the change.

❾   Corrective Action: Enter the corrective action required because of the change.

❿   Approved By: Reviewers enter your name and date when the validation change request form is complete and ready for processing.

VALIDATION CHANGE REQUEST FORM NUMBER ASSIGNMENT

The numbering systems in this part of the book are for manual paperbased documentation systems. In the paperbased system you will need logbooks to record your documentation numbers. Using logbooks allows you to see what the next available number is when you need to assign a new number. There needs to be a logbook in Document Control where validation change request form numbers are assigned (see Chapter 8 under "Validation Change Request Form Number Assignment Log").

Changes Before, During, and After Qualification Testing

Changes can be made during different time periods by using the methods shown in (Fig. 6.4). The method of changing protocol prior to qualification testing is covered in (see Chapter 4 under "Document Review and Approval"). Deviations are used to make changes to protocols during qualification testing by using a lining out

℞	**Validation Change Request Form**		
Originator:	Date:		VCRF No.: 001

Validation Baseline Affected:	Priority:
☐ Cleaning ☐ Facility ☐ Utility ☒ Equipment ☐ Computer ☐ Software ☐ Process ☐ Requal	☒ Routine ☐ Urgent

Documents Affected:

Document Number	Revision	Title
4010	C	(Any Mixer Co.) Model ME501 Emulsifying Mixer

Reason and Description of Change or (See marked-up documents):

Some of the important qualification testing was inadvertently left out of the original qualification testing.

Corrective Action:

Qualification testing will be performed and the documentation will be changed.

Approved By:

Validation Manager:	Date:
Research & Development:	Date:
Operations:	Date:
Maintenance:	Date:
Regulatory Compliance:	Date:

Form Number: V006 (5/28/98)   Reference: SOP-VAL006

method, and the deficiency form is used to notify the maintenance department that there is something wrong with the system that you are validating. Addendums are used to make changes to protocols after qualification testing and prior to certification. Changes made after the protocol has been certified are covered by using a requalification protocol (see Chapter 7).

Figure 6.4 **Protocol Change Methods**

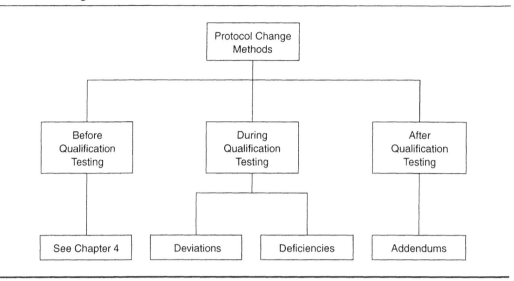

Deviation

Deviations are used to make changes to protocols during qualification testing. Why would you need to make changes to a protocol while you are performing the qualification test? If the protocol was written without pretesting the equipment there may be a difference between the protocol and the system you are validating. Another reason for a deviation would be that you discovered that you needed to change your testing approach. With a deviation, changes are made by lining out the incorrect information and entering the correct information. The changes are then initialed and dated to the right and just below all entries. The deviation will be recorded in the final report and cross referenced to its location in the protocol. (See Chapter 5 under "Final Report" for an example of how to document the deviation in the final report.) Deviations will be numbered as they occur in the protocol, then they are cross referenced in the protocol back to the final report.

Following is an example of a deviation: The original speed of a mixer was measured with a hand-held tachometer. This information was lined out, initialed, and dated, and a new measurement was taken with a calibrated remote speed controller that was specifically manufactured for the equipment.

Deficiency

The deficiency form is used to notify the maintenance department that there is something wrong with the system that you are validating. The deficiency must be resolved before the system can be certified for use. The noted deficiency in the protocol will be cross referenced to the deficiency form that will be attached to the protocol after resolution and implementation.

Deficiency Form

With this form you will be answering the following questions:

- Who prepared the deficiency form?
- What is the deficiency form number?
- What is the number and title of this system?
- What is the criticality of the deficiency?
- What departments are affected by this deficiency?
- What is the definition of the deficiency?
- What is the impact of the deficiency?
- What corrective action was taken?
- Who reviewed and approved the deficiency?

Deficiency Form Preparation

Each circled number below corresponds to the circled number on the sample deficiency form.

❶ Prepared by: Enter your name and date.

❷ DF No.: Enter the next available deficiency form number (see Chapter 8 under "Deficiency Form Number Assignment Log").

   Example: DF001

❸ System No. and Title: Enter the number and title of the system.

❹ The deficiency is: Mark the appropriate box—either "non-critical" or "critical" depending on the magnitude of the change. A non-critical deficiency would allow continued use of the system during resolution of the deficiency. A critical deficiency affects the process, thus precluding further use of the system.

❺ Affected Dept(s).: Enter the department(s) that will be affected by this change.

❻ Describe the Deficiency: Describe the deficiency in sufficient detail so that a work order can be written by the maintenance department to have the system corrected.

❼ Describe the Impact: State what impact this deficiency could have if left uncorrected.

❽ Corrective Action: Enter the corrective action that needs to be taken.

❾ Approved By: Enter your name and date when the deficiency form is forwarded to maintenance for corrective action. The maintenance signature signifies acceptance of the deficiency and that it will be acted upon.

℞	Deficiency Form		
Prepared by: ❶		Date:	DF No.: ❷
System No.: ❸ Title:			
❹ The deficiency is: Non-Critical ❑ Critical ❑			
Affected Dept(s).: ❺			
Describe the Deficiency: ❻			
Describe the impact if this deficiency is not corrected: ❼			
Corrective Action: ❽			
❾ Approved By:			
Validation:			Date:
Maintenance:			Date:

Form Number: V007 (5/28/98)   Reference: SOP-VAL007

DEFICIENCY FORM NUMBER ASSIGNMENT

There needs to be a logbook in Document Control where deficiency form numbers are assigned (see Chapter 8 under "Deficiency Form Number Assignment Log").

ADDENDUM

Addendums are used to document changes to qualification protocols after testing is complete and prior to certification approval. This is not to be confused with requalification, which comes into play after the equipment has been certified for

℞	Deficiency Form		
Prepared by:		Date: 10/17/98	DF No.: 001

System No.: 542   Title: (Any Mixer Co.) Model MX007 Matrix Mixer

The deficiency is: Non-Critical ❑ Critical ⊠

Affected Dept(s).: R&D and Operations

Describe the Deficiency: (Reference: Page 25 of Protocol 4025)

The cooling supply's water pressure was measured at 62 psig which is greater than the manufacturer's specification of ≤30 psig for the Bowl Jacket and ≤10 psig for the Washdown Valves. There is not a pressure regulator on the supply line.

Describe the impact if this deficiency is not corrected:

Blockage in the drain line could cause the water pressure in the Bowl Jacket to exceed the Jacket rating of 30 psig and the ≤10 psig for the Washdown Valves.

Corrective Action:

Work Request No. 53115 was prepared by Maintenance for corrective action. A water pressure regulator will be installed on the water supply line.

Approved By:

Validation Manager:	Date:
Maintenance:	Date:

Form Number: V007 (5/28/98)   Reference: SOP-VAL007

use. The addendum is used to clarify and/or correct information in the protocol and to add additional qualification testing. The addendum will become part of the original protocol package. This section will show you how to develop a complete addendum to a qualification protocol. The method of development applies the same to all validation department functions. You need to capture the most pertinent information that identifies which qualification addendum this is, which equipment is being validated, and who prepared and approved the addendum.

With this addendum you will be answering the following questions:

• What is the protocol number and title?

• What is the addendum number?

- Who is the equipment manufacturer?

- What is the model number and the serial number?

- What is the equipment number?

- What was the location of the equipment at the time of testing?

- Who prepared the addendum?

- Who reviewed and approved the addendum?

- Was the qualification testing successful?

Addendum – Page 1 Preparation

Each circled number below corresponds to the circled number on page 1 of the sample addendum.

❶ Protocol Number: Enter the protocol number and title (see Chapter 2 under "Protocol Numbering System" and "Title").

❷ Addendum No.: Enter the next available addendum number (see Chapter 8 under "Addendum Number Assignment Log").

Example: A001

❸ Manufacturer: Enter the name of the manufacturer.

❹ Page: Enter the page number.

Example: Page 1 of 9

This method is best for change control purposes because you will need to account for every page of the addendum.

❺ Model Number: Enter the model number.

❻ Serial Number: Enter the serial number.

❼ Equipment Number: Enter the equipment number (see Chapter 2 under "Equipment Numbering System").

Example: Minor Equipment Number: 00
            Major Equipment Number: 000

❽ Location: Enter the location of the equipment when it was tested, even if it is portable.

❾ Prepared By: Reviewers enter your name and date when the addendum is complete.

❿ Approved By: Enter your name and date when your review and approval is complete.

Addendum – Page 2

Following is an example of the second page of an addendum. You do not need to repeat the entire header on subsequent pages; you only need the information that identifies the equipment that is being

R̥	Addendum		
Protocol Number: ❶ Title:		Addendum No.: ❷	
Manufacturer: ❸		Page: ❹	
Model Number: ❺		Serial Number: ❻	
Equipment Number: ❼		Location: ❽	

Cover Page

❾	Prepared By:	
Validation:		Date:
❿	Approved By:	
Validation Manager:		Date:
Research & Development:		Date:
Operations:		Date:
Maintenance:		Date:
Regulatory Compliance:		Date:

validated, the protocol number, and the page number. Also, the footer for some of the subsequent pages is different than the footer used on page 1. On pages where entries are made, the person who performed the qualification testing will sign and date each page. The person who reviewed the completed addendum also will sign and date the addendum. There is nothing at the bottom of the page if entries were not made.

℞	Addendum	
Protocol Number: ❶	Addendum No.: ❷	
Title:	Page: ❸	

Subsequent Pages

⬎ This is only on the pages where entries are made.

Performed By: ❹	Date:
Verified By: ❺	Date:

Addendum–Page 2 Preparation

Each circled number below corresponds to the circled number on the subsequent pages of the sample addendum.

❶   Protocol Number: Enter the protocol number and title (same as page 1).

❷   Addendum No.: Enter the addendum number (same as page 1).

❸   Page: Enter the page number.

Example: Page 2 of 9

This method is best for change control purposes because you will need to account for every page of the addendum.

❹   Performed By: The person who performed the test will sign and date here. This footer only goes on the pages where entries are made.

❺   Verified By: The person who reviewed the protocol will sign and date here. This does not necessarily need to be done during qualification testing.

Completed Addendum

I have included an actual addendum template that is filled in, to show you how to develop an addendum by example. Each of the above addendum elements is covered in the template.

ADDENDUM NUMBER ASSIGNMENT

The numbering systems in this part of the book are for manual paperbased documentation systems. In the paperbased system you will need logbooks to record your documentation numbers. Using logbooks allows you to see what the next available number is when you need to assign a new number. There needs to be a logbook in Document Control where addendum numbers are assigned (see Chapter 8 under "Addendum Number Assignment Log").

℞	Addendum	
Protocol Number: 4067 Title: (Any Labeler Co.) Plastic Bottle Labeler Model 112-PB		Addendum No.: A001
Manufacturer: Any Labeler Co.		Page: 1 of 2
Model Number: 112-PB	Serial Number: 2700D79M	
Equipment Number: 245	Location: Packaging Line 9	
Prepared By:		
Validation:		Date:
Approved By:		
Validation Manager:		Date:
Research & Development:		Date:
Operations:		Date:
Maintenance:		Date:
Regulatory Compliance:		Date:

℞	**Addendum**	
Protocol Number: 4067		Addendum No.: A001
Title: (Any Labeler Co.) Plastic Bottle Labeler Model 112-PB		Page: 2 of 2

Operational Qualification

Imprinter Operation

Objective

The objective of this addendum is to add the qualification testing of the imprinter to the original validation. The imprinter was not validated because it was not ever used. It has been determined that there is a need for this function.

Method

- Visually observe 100 connective 1 3/4" x 3 3/8" size labels as they pass through imprinter and verify that 100% of the labels have a serial number and date printed on them. Record the results in the following Table I.

- Visually observe 100 connective 2 1/2" x 6" size labels as they pass through imprinter and verify that 100% of the labels have a serial number and date printed on them. Record the results in the following Table I.

Table I   Imprinter Test Results

Test	Number of Labels	Label Size	Number of Labels Imprinted	Acceptable (Yes/No)
1	100	1 3/4" x 3 3/8"	100	Yes
2	100	2 1/2" x 6"	100	Yes

Performed By:	Date:
Verified By:	Date:

Chapter 7

Requalification

This chapter covers the next logical step in the validation process, the requalification protocol. The methods that are described in this chapter apply to all of the validation department functions: cleaning, facilities, utilities, equipment, computer, software, and process. I have used the words "requal" and "requalification" throughout the book.

With requalification, the big question is: How often do you need to revalidate a system after it is validated the first time? After a certain period of time has passed, or after something has changed? What about when nothing has changed? There are at least three answers:

1. At least once a year for a system with controllers (PC, PLC, microprocessors, etc.) that is critical to the process.

2. Every 2 years for a simple system, to ensure that everything remains within a validated state of control.

3. Because something has changed.

The method that I am showing in this book is the change control method. It is more economical to incorporate a revalidation approach that is based on change, because you are not validating systems all the time. When changes are made to a baselined system, validation will need to be conducted prior to placing the system back into service (see Chapter 6).

REASONS FOR REQUALIFICATION

Following are some common reasons for requalification.

Equipment was relocated

Equipment was modified

Critical items have been replaced or repaired

Product changed

Process changed

System upgrades have been added

Computer systems have been replaced

Additions to the functionality of the system have been made

Time

A lot of changes have been made

Regulatory requirements have changed

Records were lost

REQUALIFICATION APPROACH

When a requalification protocol is required, obtain the qualification protocol package from the original time or times that the equipment was validated (see Chapter 8 under "Protocol Package Contents Sheet"). If all of the documentation was not in the package from the previous qualifications, obtain copies and add them to the new requal package. Next, identify whether all of the proper tests were performed. If not, add them to this requal protocol package. Fix any problems and update the documentation to the latest format, then compare the new results to old results for trending purposes.

Fig. 7.1 shows an example of a requal protocol, the industry tool used to document the requalification process, but it could take any form or format. During requalification testing, the performer and reviewer will sign the requal protocol at the bottom of each page where entries are made. Upon approval the requal protocol will become part of the qualification protocol package and be released into Document Control. The validation is complete when all acceptance criteria have been met. Requal protocols are test procedures, and when they are executed they become test reports. These reports are snapshots in time and are archived that way, not to be changed. I do not show a complete set of the requal protocol documents because they are the same as the qualification documents, only the word "requal" has been added.

Requal protocol attachments are created to allow for the addition of other departments' and companies' documentation, test data results, deficiencies, and batch records. The requal protocol will be written by a validation specialist and approved by the validation manager, Research and Development, Operations, Maintenance, and Regulatory Compliance. Upon approval, the requal protocol will be used to perform qualification testing, then it will become part of the requal protocol package and released into Document Control. The same format is used for requal protocols that is used for the original protocol. The idea is to have all of

Figure 7.1   ***Requal Protocol Documentation***

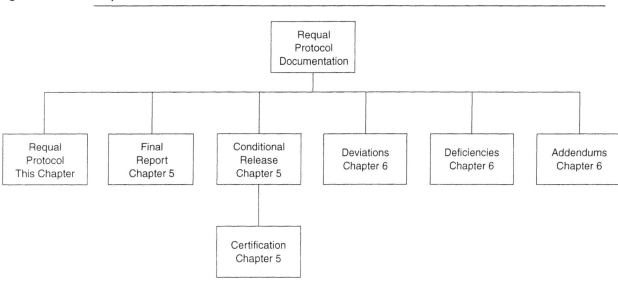

your information-gathering documents the same, as much as possible, because being repetitive is more economical. Any time you have variations you waste time and money.

REQUAL PROTOCOL

This section will show you how to develop a complete equipment requal protocol; the method of development applies the same to all validation department functions. You need to capture the most pertinent information that identifies which qualification this is, which equipment is being validated, and who prepared and approved the requal protocol. With the requal protocol you will be answering the following questions:

- What is the requal protocol title?

- What is the requal protocol number?

- Who is the equipment manufacturer?

- What is the model number and the serial number?

- What is the equipment number?

- What was the location of the equipment at the time of testing?

- Who prepared the requal protocol?

- Who reviewed and approved the requal protocol?

- Which equipment is being revalidated?

- Was the requalification testing successful?

R̥	**Equipment Requal Protocol**		
Title: ❶		Requal No.: ❷	
Manufacturer: ❸		Page: ❹	
Model Number: ❺	Serial Number: ❻		
Equipment Number: ❼	Location: ❽		
Cover Page			
❾ **Prepared By:**			
Validation:			Date:
❿ **Approved By:**			
Validation Manager:			Date:
Research & Development:			Date:
Operations:			Date:
Maintenance:			Date:
Regulatory Compliance:			Date:

Requal Protocol – Page 1 Preparation

Each circled number below corresponds to the circled number on page 1 of the sample equipment requal protocol.

❶   Title: Enter the requal protocol title (see Chapter 2 under "Protocol Title").

Example: (Any Mixer Co.) Model ME501 Emulsifying Mixer

❷   Requal No.: Enter the next available requal protocol letter (see Chapter 8 under "Protocol Number Assignment Log").

Example: 4010 C

❸   Manufacturer: Enter the name of the manufacturer.

❹   Page: Enter the page number.

> *Example:* Page 1 of 9

> This method is best for change control purposes because you will need to account for every page of the requal protocol.

❺   Model Number: Enter the model number.

❻   Serial Number: Enter the serial number.

❼   Equipment Number: Enter the equipment number (see Chapter 2 under "Equipment Numbering System").

> *Example:* Minor Equipment Number: 00
>   Major Equipment Number: 000

❽   Location: Enter the location of the equipment when it was tested, even if it is portable.

❾   Prepared By: Enter your name and date when the requal protocol is complete.

❿   Approved By: Enter your name and date when your review and approval is complete.

Requal Protocol – Page 2

Following is an example of the second page of an equipment requal protocol. You do not need to repeat the entire header on subsequent pages; you only need the information that identifies the equipment that is being validated, the requal protocol number, and the page number. Following is an example of a footer for the second page of a requal protocol. For an example of a filled-in page 2 footer, see page 2 of the completed requal protocol. The footer for the subsequent pages is different than that on page 1, because on pages where entries are made, the person who performed the qualification testing will sign and date each page. Also, the person who reviewed the completed requal protocol will sign and date the requal protocol.

Requal Protocol – Page 2 Preparation

Each circled number below corresponds to the circled number on the subsequent pages of the sample equipment requal protocol.

❶   Title: Enter the requal protocol title (same as page 1).

❷   Requal Number: Enter the requal protocol letter (same as page 1).

❸   Page Number: Enter the page number.

> *Example:* Page 2 of 9
> This method is best for change control purposes because you will need to account for every page of the requal protocol.

❹   Performed By: The person who performed the test will sign and date here. This footer only goes on the pages where entries are made.

❺   Verified By: The person who reviewed the requal protocol will sign and date here. This does not necessarily need to be done during requalification testing.

Ŗ	**Equipment Requal Protocol**		
Title: ❶		Requal No.: ❷	
		Page: ❸	

Subsequent Pages

✻ This is only on the pages where entries are made.

Performed By: ❹	Date:
Verified By: ❺	Date:

COMPLETED EQUIPMENT REQUAL PROTOCOL

Fig. 7.2 shows the major elements of an equipment requalification protocol. The requal protocol examples in this book can be used as cGMP compliance guides, and they should be tailored to meet individual company requirements. Not all of the elements that are shown will be required for each requalification. The depth of the changes will dictate the number of elements that will appear in the requal protocol.

Figure 7.2   ***Equipment Requal Protocol Contents***

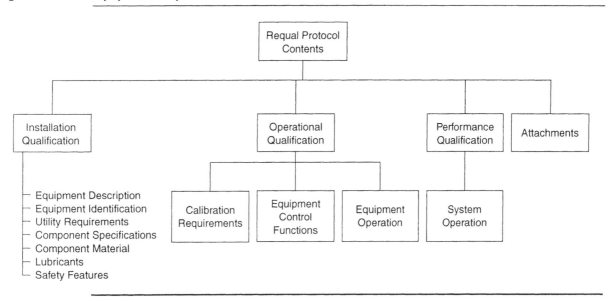

I have included an actual requal protocol template that is filled-in, thus showing you how to develop a requal protocol by example. There are several ways to document a requalification, but the one I am showing you is a user-friendly (FDA) method. This is the requalification of the same mixer that is shown in Chapter 3. In the following example the motor on that piece of equipment was changed. Therefore you will have to change only the pages that are associated with a motor change. The requal protocol will have its own page numbering system, but the sections and paragraphs that are shown in the requal protocol are taken from the original protocol.

In the following example you will see that because of the motor change, I started with the first item in the original protocol that was affected by that change. Then I went down through the original protocol and addressed the items that were affected by the change. Following is a list of items that may have been affected by the motor change and the retesting that will need to be performed.

- See if the SOPs have changed since the original validation.

- The volts and amps will have to be retested.

- The instrument used to do the testing will need to be recorded.

- The major components will have to include the new motor information.

- The lubrication will have to be checked to see if it changed.

- The motor rotation test will need to be performed.

- The motor speed test will need to be performed.

- The instrument used to measure the speed will need to be recorded.

- Calibration certificates will need to be attached to the requal protocol.

Using this method you can do a direct comparison of the original protocol and the requal protocol.

R	**Equipment Requal Protocol**		
Title: (Any Mixer Co.) Model ME501 Emulsifying Mixer		Requal No.: 4010 C	
Manufacturer: Any Mixer Co.			Page: 1 of 8
Model Number: ME 501		Serial Number: 55356 B	
Equipment Number: 2052		Location: Room 802 (This equipment is portable.)	

Prepared By:	
Validation:	Date:
Approved By:	
Validation Manager:	Date:
Research & Development:	Date:
Operations:	Date:
Maintenance:	Date:
Regulatory Compliance:	Date:

R	**Equipment Requal Protocol**	Protocol No.: 4010 C
Title: (Any Mixer Co.) Model ME501 Emulsifying Mixer		Page: 2 of 8

5.2 Required Documentation

Record the standard operating procedures that cover the setup, operation and cleaning of the mixer in Table II.

Table II Standard Operating Procedures

Number	Description	Release Date
GRA025	Granulation Equipment Setup	10/23/92
GRA026	Granulation Department Equipment Cleaning Procedure	03/12/96

5.3 Equipment Utility Requirements

Compare the manufacturer's specified volt (V) and amps (A) requirements to their as-found condition at the time of requalification testing and record the results in Table IV. Also, record the location of the power supply source. Record the instrument used to measure the volts and amps in Table V.

Volt Calculation:

Volt specification = 460 V ±10%
±10% of 460 = ±46
460 + 46 = 506
460 - 46 = 414
The measured volts of 461/468/466 fall within ±10%

Prepared By:	Date:
Verified By:	Date:

℞ **Equipment Requal Protocol**	Protocol No.: 4010 C
Title: (Any Mixer Co.) Model ME501 Emulsifying Mixer	Page: 3 of 8

Amp Calculation:

    Circuit rating = 20 A
    Equipment current draw = 12.2 A
The circuit amp rating of 20 is greater than the maximum current draw of the equipment.

Table IV   Utilities

Utility	Specified	Measured Results	Acceptable (Yes/No)
Volts	460 ±10%	A-B 461 A-C 468 B-C 466	Yes
Amps	Motor = 12.2	20 Circuit Rating	Yes

Power supply source, breaker box BB1, wire numbers: 31, 33, 35.

Table V   Instrument Used

Test Instrument	Identification Number	Calibration Due Date
Multimeter	ME-025	04/19/97

5.4   Major Component Specifications

The section is used to verify that the mixer components purchased were delivered and installed. Record the major components in Table VI.

Prepared By:	Date:
Verified By:	Date:

R̸ Equipment Requal Protocol	Protocol No.: 4010 C
Title: (Any Mixer Co.) Model ME501 Emulsifying Mixer	Page: 4 of 8

Table VI   Major Components

Components	As-found Conditions
Mixer Motor	Manufacturer: Any Motor Co. Model Number: ME 501 Serial Number: 55356 C Volts: 460 Amperes: 12.2 Phases: 3 Cycles: 60 Hz hp: 5 rpm: 3480

5.6   Lubricants

Record the lubricant used to operate the mixer in Table VII and indicate if they make contact with the product. Is there is a preventive maintenance procedure on file? (Yes/No) *Yes*

Table VII   Lubricants

Where Used	Type	Manufacturer	Product Contact (Yes/No)
Motor Bearings	Lubriplate 630 AA	Any Oil Co.	No

Prepared By:	Date:
Verified By:	Date:

℞ **Equipment Requal Protocol**	Protocol No.: 4010 C

Title: (Any Mixer Co.) Model ME501 Emulsifying Mixer	Page: 5 of 8

6.3   Equipment Operation

6.3.1   Mixer Rotation Direction Test

Test Objective. The objective of this test is to verify that the mixer motor rotates in the proper direction. The mixer will be operated with the impeller being submerged in water.

Test Procedure

Materials and instruments required: mixing container, test fluid

- Fill the mixing container with water to its maximum working volume of 103 L and record the amount used in Table XII. When operating the mixer the head must be submerged in the water to prevent damage to the mixer.

  Test fluid volume calculation:

  Test fluid volume = 75% of 138 L = 103.5 L (rounded off to 103 L)

- Press the Start key and observe the direction of rotation of the mixer motor as viewed from the top of the mixer and record the results in Table XIII.

Table XII   Test Materials

Item	Results
Mixing Container	138 L
Test Fluid	Water
Test Fluid Volume	103 L

Prepared By:	Date:
Verified By:	Date:

Ŗ	**Equipment Requal Protocol**	Protocol No.: 4010 C

Title: (Any Mixer Co.) Model ME501 Emulsifying Mixer	Page: 6 of 8

Table XIII   Mixer Motor Rotation Direction Test Results

Item	Expected Results	Results	Acceptable (Yes/No)
Mixer Motor Rotation Direction	Rotation should be clockwise as viewed from the top of the mixer.	Clockwise rotation was observed.	Yes

7.1   Emulsifying Mixer Operation

Test Objective. The objective of this test is to document the speed of the mixer motor to verify that the new motor was equivalent the old motor.

Test Procedure

Materials and instruments required: mixing container, test fluid, tachometer

- Fill the mixing container with water to its maximum working volume of 103 L. When operating the mixer the head must be submerged in the water to prevent damage to the mixer.

Test Fluid Volume Calculation:

Test fluid volume = 75% of 138 L = 103.5 L (rounded off to 103 L)

Prepared By:	Date:
Verified By:	Date:

R	**Equipment Requal Protocol**	Protocol No.: 4010 C

Title: (Any Mixer Co.) Model ME501 Emulsifying Mixer	Page: 7 of 8

- Measure the speed of the mixer with a calibrated tachometer. Verify that the measured speed is within ±10% of the fixed speed of 3480 rpm. Record the results in Table XIV and the instrument used to measure the speed in Table XV.

Mixer Speed Calculation:

Mixer speed specification = 3480 rpm ±10%
±10% of 3480 = ± 348
3480 + 348 = 3828
3480 - 348 = 3132
The measured rpm of 3521 falls within ±10%

Table XIV   Mixer Speed Test Results

Item	Specification rpm	Measured Speed rpm	Acceptable (Yes/No)
Mixer Speed	3480 ±10%	3521	Yes

Table XV   Instrument Used

Test Instrument	Identification Number	Calibration Due Date
Tachometer	64020	06/21/97

Prepared By:	Date:
Verified By:	Date:

℞	**Equipment Requal Protocol**	Protocol No.: 4010 C
Title: (Any Mixer Co.) Model ME501 Emulsifying Mixer		Page: 8 of 8

Attachment 1

Equipment Critical Instruments and
Test Equipment Calibration Certifications

Chapter 8

Document Control

This chapter covers the next logical step in the validation process, document control. Several subjects are covered in this chapter, including protocol package contents sheet, block number assignment, logbooks, document master list, and forms control. After the protocol final report has been written and approved it is time to release the complete qualification package into Document Control. Document Control has to be a department outside of Validation, because if it is not, it is like having the fox watch the hen house. Having Document Control outside of Validation gives the FDA warm fuzzies. Following are methods that you can use to have a good interface with Document Control and to make sure that you are controlling all of your validation documentation.

PROTOCOL PACKAGE CONTENTS SHEET

A protocol package contents sheet should reside on top of each protocol package that is released into Document Control. The methods that are described in this section apply to all validation department functions: cleaning, facilities, utilities, equipment, computer, software, and process. With this protocol package contents sheet you will be answering the following questions:

- What is the equipment's name?
- What is the protocol package contents sheet number?
- What is the equipment number, model number, and serial number?
- Which documents are included in the qualification package?

℞	**Protocol Package Contents Sheet**				
Equipment Name: ❶				PPCS No.: ❷	
Equipment No.: ❸	Model No.: ❹		Serial No.: ❺	Included:	
Document Number	Description			Yes	No
❻	❼			❽	

Form Number: V008 (5/28/98)   Reference: SOP-VAL008

Protocol Package Contents Sheet Preparation

Each circled number below corresponds to the circled number on the sample protocol package contents sheet.

❶   Equipment Name: Enter the name of the equipment.

❷   PPCS No.: Enter the next available protocol package contents sheet number (see page 158, under "Protocol Package Contents Sheet Number Assignment Log").

❸   Equipment No.: Enter the equipment number.

❹   Model No.: Enter the model number.

❺   Serial No.: Enter the serial number.

❻   Document Number: Enter all of the protocol and referenced documents that are in this qualification package, starting with the protocol number.

❼   Description: Enter the description of each included document.

❽   Included: Mark either "yes" or "no".

℞	**Protocol Package Contents Sheet**			
Equipment Name: *TURBULA SHAKER MIXER*				
Equipment No.: *4010*	Model No.: *MC501*	Serial No.: *55356 B*	Included:	
Number	**Description**		**Yes**	**No**
CF001	Certification, Equipment		✔	
FR001	Final Report		✔	
4010	Protocol		✔	
	Capitol App. Request			✔
	Quote			✔
	Purchase Requisition			✔
0121577	Purchase Order		✔	
8110	Invoice		✔	
	Packing Slip			✔
No number	Vendor Spec Sheet		✔	
No number	Vendor Catalog: Emulsifying Mixer		✔	
No number	Equipment Manual: Installation and Operation		✔	
00862 00871	Main Drive Drawing Control System Drawing		✔	
GRA025	SOP: Granulation Equipment Setup		✔	
No number	Engineering Standard:		✔	
No number	Preventive Maint Schedule: Monthly and 6 months		✔	
MTE-012	Calibration Certificates- Equipment Critical Instruments: MTE-FACILITIES		✔	
ME-025	Calibration Certificates-Test Instrument Multimeter		✔	
etc.				

Form Number: V008 (5/28/98)   Reference: SOP-VAL008

Block Number Assignment

All of the numbers in this book came from the following blocks of numbers. These blocks of numbers were established prior to assigning numbers to documents. This method controls the number assignment effort so that there will not be any duplicate numbers on documentation.

Equipment Numbers	
Number	**Description**
01 thru 99	Minor Equipment
001 thru 999	Major Equipment
0001 thru 9999	Validation Not Required Equipment

Protocol Numbers	
Number	**Description**
1000 thru 1999	Cleaning Validation
2000 thru 2999	Facilities Validation
3000 thru 3999	Utilities Validation
4000 thru 4999	Equipment Validation
5000 thru 5999	Computer Validation
6000 thru 6999	Software Validation
7000 thru 7999	Process Validation

Request For Validation Numbers	
Number	**Description**
RFV000 thru RFV999	Request For Validation Form

Document Review Form Numbers	
Number	**Description**
DRF000 thru DRF999	Document Review Form

Final Report Numbers	
Number	**Description**
FR000 thru FR999	Final Report

Conditional Release Form Numbers	
Number	**Description**
CRF000 thru CRF999	Conditional Release Form

Certification Form Numbers	
Number	**Description**
CF000 thru CF999	Certification Form

Validation Baseline Document Numbers	
Number	**Description**
VBD000 thru VBD999	Validation Baseline Document

Validation Change Request Form Numbers	
Number	**Description**
VCRF000 thru VCRF999	Validation Change Request Form

Deficiency Form Numbers	
Number	**Description**
DF000 thru DF999	Deficiency Form

Addendum Numbers	
Number	**Description**
A000 thru A999	Addendum

Form Numbers	
Number	**Description**
V000 thru V999	Forms

LOGBOOKS

This section includes all of the document number assignment logbooks for the entire validation documentation system. Following is a list of all of the logbooks detailed in this section.

- Equipment Number Assignment Log

- Protocol Number Assignment Log

- Request for Validation Form Number Assignment Log

- Document Review Form Number Assignment Log

- Final Report Number Assignment Log

- Conditional Release Form Number Assignment Log

- Certification Form Number Assignment Log

- Validation Baseline Document Number Assignment Log

- Validation Change Request Form Number Assignment Log

- Deficiency Form Number Assignment Log

- Addendum Number Assignment Log

- Protocol Package Contents Sheet Number Assignment Log

- Form Number Assignment Log

EQUIPMENT NUMBER ASSIGNMENT LOG

Equipment numbers are assigned in random order in the Equipment Number Assignment Log. The best method of obtaining the next available equipment number is by having a separate sheet for each of the three types of equipment numbers (00, 000, 0000). This way you can always see what the next available number is. Each of the separate logs can be loaded into a spreadsheet for sorting purposes (see Chapter 2 under "Equipment Master List"). With this log you will be answering the following questions:

- What is the equipment number?

- What is the serial number?

Ŗ̣ Equipment Number Assignment Log						
Equip. No.	Serial Number	Description	Location /Room	Reason Not Validated	Initials	Date
❶	❷	❸	❹	❺	❻	❼

- What is the description of the equipment?
- What is the location of the equipment?
- What is the reason for not validating the equipment?
- Who checked out the number?
- When was the number checked out?

Equipment Number Assignment Log Preparation

Each circled number below corresponds to the circled number on the sample Equipment Number Assignment Log.

❶   Equip. No: Enter the equipment number (see Chapter 2 under "Equipment Numbering System").

Example: 00, 000, or 0000

❷   Serial Number: Enter the serial number of the equipment.

Example: B56943

❸   Description: Enter the description of the equipment (see Chapter 2 under "Equipment Description").

Example: Talboy Model 134-2 T-line Stirrer

❹   Location/Room: Enter the location of the equipment at the time of validation.

❺   Reason Not Validated: Enter the reason why the equipment does not need to be validated, (if applicable).

Example: calibrated, utensil, or instrument

❻   Initials: Enter your initials.

❼   Date: Enter the date that the number was checked out.

PROTOCOL NUMBER ASSIGNMENT LOG

Numbers are assigned in random order in the Protocol Number Assignment Log. The best method of obtaining the next available number is by having a separate sheet for each of the major number series (1000 through 7000). This way you can always see what the next available number is. Each of the separate logs can be loaded into a spreadsheet for sorting purposes (see Chapter 2 under "Protocol Master List"). With this log you will be answering the following questions:

*   What is the qualification or requalification protocol number?
*   What is the description of the document?
*   What is the equipment number (if any)?
*   What is the serial number (if applicable)?
*   What is the location of the equipment at the time of validation (if applicable)?
*   Who produced the document?
*   When was the document completed?

℞	Equipment Number Assignment Log					
Equip. No.	Serial Number	Description	Location /Room	Reason Not Validated	Initials	Date
01	12A289	C.E. Tyler Rotap Sieve Shaker	212	N/A	PAC	08/21/98
02	85126	Groen Steam Kettle	216	N/A	PAC	08/21/98
03	etc.					
04						
05						
06						
07						
08						
09						
10						
11						
12						
13						
14						
15						
16						
17						
18						
19						
20						
21						

Log page for the major equipment three-digit numbers.

℞	**Equipment Number Assignment Log**					
Equip. No.	**Serial Number**	**Description**	**Location /Room**	**Reason Not Validated**	**Initials**	**Date**
001	I6613	Stokes Rd-3(D) Tablet Press	652	N/A	PAC	08/21/98
002	85126	Groen Steam Kettle	Dev Lab	N/A	PAC	08/21/98
003	etc.					
004						
005						
006						
007						
008						
009						
010						
011						
012						
013						
014						
015						
016						
017						
018						
019						
020						
021						

Log page for the validation not required four-digit numbers.

℞	Equipment Number Assignment Log					
Equip. No.	Serial Number	Description	Location /Room	Reason Not Validated	Initials	Date
0001	B5694	Mettler Model AE100 Precision Balance	Dev Lab	Calibrated	PAC	08/21/98
0002	85126	Talboy Model 134-2 T-line Stirrer	Dev Lab	Utensil	PAC	08/21/98
0003	etc.					
0004						
0005						
0006						
0007						
0008						
0009						
0010						
0011						
0012						
0013						
0014						
0015						
0016						
0017						
0018						
0019						
0020						

℞	Protocol Number Assignment Log					
Protocol Number	**Description**	**Equip. No.**	**Serial No.**	**Location /Room**	**Initials**	**Com. Date**
❶	❷	❸	❹	❺	❻	❼

Protocol Number Assignment Log Preparation

Each circled number below corresponds to the circled number on the sample Protocol Number Assignment Log.

❶   Protocol Number: Enter the qualification or requalification protocol number (see Chapter 2 under "Protocol Numbering System").

Example: 7006 (process validation new protocol number)

❷   Description: Enter the document description (see Chapter 2 under "Protocol Title").

Example: (Product Name) USP 600/150 mg, 4 M

❸   Equipment No.: Enter the equipment number, if applicable.

❹   Serial No.: Enter the serial number, if applicable.

❺   Location/Room: Enter the location of the equipment at the time of validation, if applicable.

❻   Initials: Enter your initials.

❼   Com. Date: Enter the date when the document is complete (released into Document Control).

℞	**Protocol Number Assignment Log**						
Protocol Number	**Description**	**Equip. No.**	**Serial No.**	**Location /Room**	**Initials**	**Com. Date**
1001	Equipment Cleaning of (Product Name)	-	-	275	PAC	01/24/98
1002	Equipment Cleaning of (Product Name)	-	-	276	PAC	06/15/98
1003	etc.					
1004						
1005						
1006						
1007						
1008						
1009						
1010						
1011						
1012						
1013						
1014						
1015						
1016						
1017						
1018						
1019						
1020						
1021						

Log page for the 2000 number series Facilities Validation protocol or requal numbers.

℞	**Protocol Number Assignment Log**					
Protocol Number	**Description**	**Equip. No.**	**Serial No.**	**Location /Room**	**Initials**	**Com. Date**
2001	Production Room 147 Qualification	-	-	147	PAC	02/02/98
2002	Production Room 275 Qualification	-	-	300	PAC	07/14/98
2003	etc.					
2004						
2005						
2006						
2007						
2008						
2009						
2010						
2011						
2012						
2013						
2014						
2015						
2016						
2017						
2018						
2019						
2020						
2021						

Log page for the 3000 number series Utilities Validation protocol and requal numbers.

R	Protocol Number Assignment Log					
Protocol Number	Description	Equip. No.	Serial No.	Location /Room	Initials	Com. Date
3001	Distilled Water System, QA Laboratory	125	Y3417	QC Lab	PAC	03/24/98
3002	Steam Generator	456	SG16	Ops	PAC	4/22/98
3003	etc.					
3004						
3005						
3006						
3007						
3008						
3009						
3010						
3011						
3012						
3013						
3014						
3015						
3016						
3017						
3018						
3019						
3020						
3021						

Log page for the 4000 number series Equipment Validation protocol and requal numbers.

℞	Protocol Number Assignment Log					
Protocol Number	Description	Equip. No.	Serial No.	Location /Room	Initials	Com. Date
4001	Compu-Coat 4 Tablet Coating Machine	864	CP001	356	PAC	04/17/98
4002	PMA-65-2G Matrix, Mixer	322	MM11	267	PAC	12/16/98
4003	etc.					
4004						
4005						
4006						
4007						
4008						
4009						
4010						
4011						
4012						
4013						
4014						
4015						
4016						
4017						
4018						
4019						
4020						

Log page for the 5000 number series Computer Validation protocol and requal numbers.

℞	Protocol Number Assignment Log						
Protocol Number	**Description**	**Equip. No.**	**Serial No.**	**Location /Room**	**Initials**	**Com. Date**
5001	Datamyte Addendum 2, Version 1.1-R&D	534	BM00	479	PAC	05/28/98
5002	Automated Weigh and Dispense System	388	AW33	562	PAC	10/24/98
5003	etc.					
5004						
5005						
5006						
5007						
5008						
5009						
5010						
5011						
5012						
5013						
5014						
5015						
5016						
5017						
5018						
5019						
5020						
5021						

Log page for the 6000 number series Software Validation protocol and requal numbers.

R	Protocol Number Assignment Log					
Protocol Number	Description	Equip. No.	Serial No.	Location /Room	Initials	Com. Date
6001	AS400 System Software	-	-	-	PAC	06/10/98
6002	DDP.WR1 Symphony Worksheet	-	-	-	PAC	04/30/98
6003	etc.					
6004						
6005						
6006						
6007						
6008						
6009						
6010						
6011						
6012						
6013						
6014						
6015						
6016						
6017						
6018						
6019						
6020						

Log page for the 7000 number series Process Validation protocol and requal numbers.

Ṛ	Protocol Number Assignment Log					
Protocol Number	Description	Equip. No.	Serial No.	Location /Room	Initials	Com. Date
7001	(Product Name) USP 300/30 mg, 2.8 M	-	-	-	PAC	3/29/98
7002	(Product Name) USP 600/150, 4 M	-	-	-	PAC	5/12/98
7003	etc.					
7004						
7005						
7006						
7007						
7008						
7009						
7010						
7011						
7012						
7013						
7014						
7015						
7016						
7017						
7018						
7019						
7020						
7021						

REQUEST FOR VALIDATION FORM NUMBER ASSIGNMENT LOG

Numbers are assigned in random order in the Request for Validation Form Number Assignment Log. Using a log such as this enables easy identification of the next available number (see Chapter 2 under "Request for Validation Form"). With this log you will be answering the following questions:

- What is the request for validation form number?
- What is the description of the system?
- Who checked out the number?
- When was the number checked out?

Request for Validation Form Number Assignment Log Preparation

Each circled number below corresponds to the circled number on the sample Request for Validation Form Number Assignment Log.

❶ RFV Number: Enter the next request for validation form number.

Example: RFV001

❷ Description: Enter the system description.

❸ Initials: Enter your initials.

❹ Date: Enter the date that the number was checked out.

DOCUMENT REVIEW FORM NUMBER ASSIGNMENT LOG

Numbers are assigned in random order in the Document Review Form Number Assignment Log. Using a log such as this enables easy identification of the next available number (see Chapter 4 under "Document Review Form"). With this log you will be answering the following questions.

- What is the document review form number?
- What is the description of the system?
- Who checked out the number?
- When was the number checked out?

Document Review Form Number Assignment Log Preparation

Each circled number below corresponds to the circled number on the sample Document Review Form Number Assignment Log.

❶ DRF Number: Enter the next document review form number.

Example: DRF001

❷ Description: Enter the system description.

❸ Initials: Enter your initials.

❹ Date: Enter the date that the number was checked out.

℞ Request For Validation Form No. Assignment Log			
RFV Number	Description	Initials	Date
❶	❷	❸	❹

FINAL REPORT NUMBER ASSIGNMENT LOG

Numbers are assigned in random order in the Final Report Number Assignment Log. Using a log such as this enables easy identification of the next available number. With this log you will be answering the following questions:

- What is the final report number?
- What is the description of the system?

℞ Document Review Form Number Assignment Log			
DRF Number	Description	Initials	Date
❶	❷	❸	❹

- Who checked out the number?
- When was the number checked out?

Final Report Number Assignment Log Preparation

Each circled number below corresponds to the circled number on the sample Final Report Number Assignment Log.

℞	Final Report Number Assignment Log			
FR Number	Description	Initials	Date	
❶	❷	❸	❹	

❶   FR Number: Enter the next final report number.

Example: FR001

❷   Description: Enter the system description.

❸   Initials: Enter your initials.

❹   Date: Enter the date that the number was checked out.

Conditional Release Form Number Assignment Log

Numbers are assigned in random order in the Conditional Release Form Number Assignment Log. Using a log such as this enables easy identification of the next available number. With this log you will be answering the following questions:

- What is the conditional release form number?
- What is the description of the system?
- Who checked out the number?
- When was the number checked out?

Conditional Release Form Number Assignment Log Preparation

Each circled number below corresponds to the circled number on the sample Conditional Release Form Number Assignment Log.

❶ CRF Number: Enter the next conditional release form number.

Example: CRF001

❷ Description: Enter the system description.

❸ Initials: Enter your initials.

❹ Date: Enter the date that the number was checked out.

Certification Form Number Assignment Log

Numbers are assigned in random order in the Certification Form Number Assignment Log. Using a log such as this enables easy identification of the next available number. With this log you will be answering the following questions:

- What is the certification form number?
- What is the description of the system?
- Who checked out the number?
- When was the number checked out?

Certification Form Number Assignment Log Preparation

Each circled number below corresponds to the circled number on the sample Certification Form Number Assignment Log.

❶ CF Number: Enter the next certification form number.

Example: CF001

❷ Description: Enter the system description.

❸ Initials: Enter your initials.

❹ Date: Enter the date that the number was checked out.

R̶ **Conditional Release Form Number Assignment Log**			
CRF Number	Description	Initials	Date
❶	❷	❸	❹

VALIDATION BASELINE DOCUMENT NUMBER ASSIGNMENT LOG

Numbers are assigned in random order in the Validation Baseline Document Number Assignment Log. Using a log such as this enables easy identification of the next available number . With this log you will be answering the following questions:

- What is the validation baseline document number?

- What is the description of the system?

℞	Certification Form Number Assignment Log			
CF Number	Description		Initials	Date
❶	❷		❸	❹

- Who checked out the number?
- When was the number checked out?

Validation Baseline Document Number Assignment Log Preparation

Each circled number below corresponds to the circled number on the sample Validation Baseline Document Number Assignment Log.

R Validation Baseline Document No. Assignment Log			
VBD Number	Description	Initials	Date
❶	❷	❸	❹

❶   VBD Number: Enter the next validation baseline document number.

Example: VBD001

❷   Description: Enter the system description.

❸   Initials: Enter your initials.

❹   Date: Enter the date that the number was checked out.

Validation Change Request Form Number Assignment Log

Numbers are assigned in random order in the Validation Change Request Form Number Assignment Log. Using a log such as this enables easy identification of the next available number. With this log you will be answering the following questions:

- What is the validation change request form number?

- What is the description of the system?

- Who checked out the number?

- When was the number checked out?

Validation Change Request Form Number Assignment Log Preparation

Each circled number below corresponds to the circled number on the sample Validation Change Request Form Number Assignment Log.

❶ VCRF Number: Enter the next validation change request form number.

Example: VCRF001

❷ Description: Enter the system description.

❸ Initials: Enter your initials.

❹ Date: Enter the date that the number was checked out.

Deficiency Form Number Assignment Log

Numbers are assigned in random order in the Deficiency Form Number Assignment Log. Using a log such as this enables easy identification of the next available number. With this log you will be answering the following questions:

- What is the deficiency form number?

- What is the description of the system?

- Who checked out the number?

- When was the number checked out?

Deficiency Form Number Assignment Log Preparation

Each circled number below corresponds to the circled number on the sample Deficiency Form Number Assignment Log.

❶ DF Number: Enter the next deficiency form number.

Example: DF001

❷ Description: Enter the system description.

❸ Initials: Enter your initials.

❹ Date: Enter the date that the number was checked out.

℞ Validation Change Request Form No. Assignment Log			
VCRF Number	Description	Initials	Date
❶	❷	❸	❹

ADDENDUM NUMBER ASSIGNMENT LOG

Numbers are assigned in random order in the Addendum Number Assignment Log. Using a log such as this enables easy identification of the next available number. With this log you will be answering the following questions:

- What is the addendum number?
- What is the description of the system?

℞	Deficiency Form Number Assignment Log		
DF Number	Description	Initials	Date
❶	❷	❸	❹

- Who checked out the number?
- When was the number checked out?

Addendum Number Assignment Log Preparation

Each circled number below corresponds to the circled number on the sample Addendum Number Assignment Log.

℞	Addendum Number Assignment Log		
Addendum Number	Description	Initials	Date
❶	❷	❸	❹

❶   Addendum Number: Enter the next addendum number.

Example: A001

❷   Description: Enter the system description.

❸   Initials: Enter your initials.

❹   Date: Enter the date that the number was checked out.

PROTOCOL PACKAGE CONTENTS SHEET NUMBER ASSIGNMENT LOG

Numbers are assigned in random order in the Protocol Package Contents Sheet Number Assignment Log. Using a log such as this eanbles easy identification of the next available number. With this log you will be answering the following questions:

- What is the protocol package contents sheet number?

- What is the description of the system?

- Who checked out the number?

- When was the number checked out?

Protocol Package Contents Sheet Number Assignment Log Preparation

Each circled number below corresponds to the circled number on the sample Protocol Package Contents Sheet Number Assignment Log.

❶   PPCS Number: Enter the next protocol package contents sheet number.

Example: PPCS001

❷   Description: Enter the system description.

❸   Initials: Enter your initials.

❹   Date: Enter the date that the number was checked out.

FORM NUMBER ASSIGNMENT LOG

Numbers are assigned in random order in the Form Number Assignment Log. Using a log such as this enables easy identification of the next available number. With this log you will be answering the following questions:

- What is the form number?

- What is the description of the form?

- Who checked out the number?

- When was the number checked out?

Form Number Assignment Log Preparation

Each circled number below corresponds to the circled number on the sample Form Number Assignment Log.

❶   Form Number: Enter the next form number.

Example: V001

❷   Description: Enter the system description.

❸   Initials: Enter your initials.

❹   Date: Enter the date that the number was checked out.

R Protocol Package Contents Sheet No. Assignment Log			
PPCS Number	Description	Initials	Date
❶	❷	❸	❹

℞	Form Number Assignment Log			
Form Number	Description		Initials	Date
❶	❷		❸	❹

R̶	Form Number Assignment Log		
Form Number	**Description**	**Initials**	**Date**
V001	Request for Validation Form	PAC	5/28/98
V002	Document Review Form	PAC	5/28/98
V003	Conditional Release Form	PAC	5/28/98
V004	Certification Form	PAC	5/28/98
V005	Validation Baseline Document	PAC	5/28/98
V006	Validation Change Request Form	PAC	5/28/98
V007	Deficiency Form	PAC	5/28/98
V008	Protocol Package Contents Sheet	PAC	5/28/98

DOCUMENT MASTER LIST

After the protocols are released into Document Control you will need to establish a Document Master List. This list will show all of the protocol documentation. This is the key spreadsheet that is used to identify which documents are filed in Document Control. The validation documentation master list will cover all of the validation department functions: facilities, utilities, equipment, computer, software, and process. With this list you will be answering the following questions:

- What is the protocol number?

- What is the description of the document?

- What is the equipment number (if any)?

- What is the serial number (if applicable)?

- What is the location of the equipment at the time of validation (if applicable)

- Who produced the document?

- When was the document released into document control?

Document Master List Preparation

Each circled number below corresponds to the circled number on the sample document master list.

❶   Protocol Number: Enter the protocol numbers to the right.

❷   Documents: Enter all of the numbers of the associated documentation below the applicable protocol.

FORMS CONTROL

If your forms are not an integral part of your procedures they will need to have a cross-reference system with the procedures. Notice at the bottom of the following example form that the form number is cross-referenced to the procedure (the form number is V006 and the procedure number is VAL006). As with other document numbers, form numbers should be assigned through a logbook in Document Control.

R	Document Master List			
Protocol Number ⇨	**❶**			
Documents　❷				
Title				
Equipment Number				
Serial Number				
Location/Room				
Request For Validation No.				
Final Report No.				
Conditional Release No.				
Certification No.				
Validation Baseline Document No.				
Validation Change Request Form Number				
Deficiency Form Number				
Addendum Number				
Protocol Package Contents Sheet Number				
Initials				
Document Control Date				
Etc.				

℞ Document Master List				
Protocol Number ⇨	4010	4011	4012	4013
Title	Mixer	Labeler		
Equipment Number	345	RFV001		
Serial Number	78129	FR001		
Location/Room	500	CRF001		
Request For Validation No.	RFV001	CF001		
Final Report No.	FR001	VBD001		
Conditional Release No.	CRF001	VCR001		
Certification No.	CF001	DF001		
Validation Baseline Document No.	VBD001	A001		
Validation Change Request Form Number	VCR001	PPCS001		
Deficiency Form Number	DF001	PAC		
Addendum Number	A001	08/28/98		
Protocol Package Contents Sheet Number	PPCS001	PPCS002		
Initials	PAC	PAC		
Document Control Date	08/28/98	08/30/98		
Etc.				

℞	**Validation Change Request Form**	
Originator:	Date:	VCRF No.:

Validation Baseline Affected:	Priority:
☐ Cleaning ☐ Facility ☐ Utility ☒ Equipment	☒ Routine ☐ Urgent
☐ Computer ☐ Software ☐ Process ☐ Requal	

Documents Affected:		
Document Number	Revision	Title
4010	C	(Any Mixer Co.) Model ME501 Emulsifying Mixer

Reason and Description of Change or (See marked-up documents):

Some of the important qualification testing was inadvertently left out of the original qualification testing.

Corrective Action:

Qualification testing will be performed and the documentation will be changed.

Approved By:	
Validation Manager:	Date:
Research & Development:	Date:
Operations:	Date:
Maintenance:	Date:
Regulatory Compliance:	Date:

Form Number: V006 (5/28/98)   Reference: SOP-VAL006

Chapter 9

Electronic Documentation Database

PROTOCOL NUMBER STRUCTURE

This chapter shows an electronic method of assigning document numbers and establishing an electronic database. The method detailed in Chapter 2 is for a manual paperbased documentation system. All qualification protocols need to have a unique number and name assigned to them for identification and tracking purposes. The protocol number is used as a locator (find number) in a database, and identifies the department function that owns the protocol and whether it is an initial qualification or a requalification. Also, the protocol number is used to identify all of the protocol's associated documentation such as certifications, final reports, deficiencies, and addendums. A complete qualification protocol identification number is made up of a prefix, base number, and suffix (see Fig. 9.1).

Qualification and Requalification Protocol Number Structure

This number structure allows you to identify which department the protocol belongs to and it uniquely identifies each qualification or requalification protocol.
Number Example: CL005-02.D01

CL = Prefix

005-02 = Base number

D01 = Suffix

Prefix

The prefix part of the protocol number is based on the first letter of each of the validation department functions and the word "validation". When the protocol master list

167

Figure 9.1   **Protocol Number Structure**

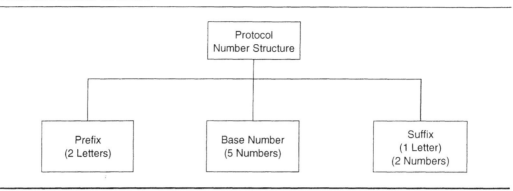

is sorted off of these letters they are grouped by department function. "CL" was used for "cleaning validation" because "CV" is used for computer validation.

CL   =   Cleaning

FV   =   Facilities

UV   =   Utilities

EV   =   Equipment

CV   =   Computer

SV   =   Software

PV   =   Process

Base Number

The base number contains two parts. The first three digits are reserved for protocol numbers and the second two digits are for requal protocol numbers. This system allows for:

000 to 999 different qualification protocols
99 requalifications to each original protocol

Suffix

The suffix contains two-parts. The letters represent the protocol's associated documents and the two-digit number allows for 99 of those documents. For example, A00 through A99 allows for 99 addendums.

A00 = Addendum

C00 = Certification

D00 = Deficiency

F00 = Final report

Figure 9.2   **Associated Documentation**

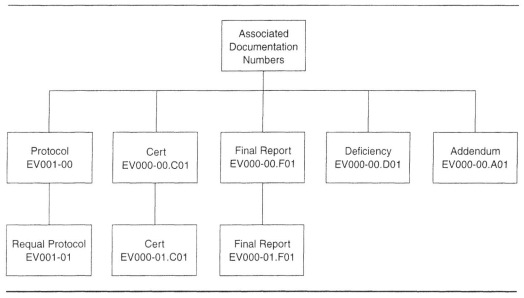

Identification Numbers And Interpretation

Complete Number	Interpretation
CV000-00.D01	This would be the first deficiency to the original computer qualification protocol.
CV000-00.D02	This would be the second deficiency to the original computer qualification protocol.
CV000-01.D01	This would be the first deficiency to the first computer requal protocol.
CV000-01.D02	This would be the second deficiency to the first computer requal protocol.
FV025-09	This would be the ninth requal of the 25th protocol.
FV025-09.A01	This would be the first addendum to the ninth requal protocol of the 25th protocol.

ASSOCIATED DOCUMENTATION NUMBERS

The above protocol numbering system provides a method for tying all of the protocol's documentation into a single package that can be used for filing and retrieving and FDA audits. This is where the base number comes into play. All of the numbers in Fig. 9.2 have one set of numbers in common. The three-digit number after the two-letter prefix is the same for the protocol and all of its associated documentation.

Table 9.1 shows what a qualification protocol numbering system might look like over time. The initial qualification protocol has one addendum, one certification,

Table 9.1 **Protocol Number Development Over Time**

Protocol Identification Numbers	
Computer Find Number	*Document Type*
Initial Qualification	
EV001-00	Protocol
EV001-00.A01	First addendum
EV001-00.C01	Certification
EV001-00.D01	First deficiency
EV001-00.D02	Second deficiency
EV001-00.D03	Third deficiency
EV001-00.F01	Final report
First Requal	
EV001-01	Protocol
EV001-01.C01	Certification
EV001-01.D01	First deficiency
EV001-01.D02	Second deficiency
EV001-01.F01	Final report
Second Requal	
EV001-02	Protocol
EV001-02.C01	Certification
EV001-02.D01	First deficiency
EV001-02.F01	Final report
Etc.	

three deficiencies, and a final report written against it. The first requal has one certification, two deficiencies, and a final report. The second requal has one certification, one deficiency, and a final report written against it. There will always be just one certification and one final report, but there may be several addendums and deficiencies written against the same protocol or requal protocol.

PROTOCOL NAMES

The protocol name is the most important locator in a database because people always remember a name long before they remember a number. You will be

Table 9.2	*Titles Sorted in Alphabetical Order*
	Tablet Press, Fette-Model 2090
	Tablet Press, Fette-Model 3090
	Tablet Press, Manesty Unipress-34 Station
	Tablet Press, Stokes-RD-3 (D)

naming your protocols so that you can easily identify which system was validated just by reading the title. The protocol title will be the same as the system description plus a few modifiers. The name will have to follow a set pattern— for equipment it would be Tablet Press, Fette-Model 2090. This is called the noun-phrase method, the noun being "tablet press" and the phrase being the manufacturer's name and model number and/or any other identifying information so that you can distinguish between different pieces of equipment. This method is used so that you can sort the document database by systems. This naming method allows you to group similar systems next to each other in the database (Table 9.2).

Equipment noun-phrase method:

Tablet Press, Fette-Model 2090

The above example reads like this: Fette Model 2090 Tablet Press.

DOCUMENT DATABASE

You will need to identify which protocols need to be written by establishing a document database. The list will show all of the protocol, addendum, certification, deficiency, and final report numbers. This is the key database that is used for planning, scheduling, and status of all validation projects. The document database is used for identifying the latest document number that was assigned for each type of document. The validation documentation database will cover all of the validation department functions: facilities, utilities, equipment, computer, software, and process. With this list you will be answering the following questions:

- What is the document number?
- What is the description of the document?
- What is the equipment number (if any)?
- What is the serial number (if applicable)?
- What is the location of the equipment at the time of validation (if applicable)?
- Who produced the document?
- When was the document completed?

℞	Document Database						
Document Number	Description	Equip. No.	Serial No.	Location	Initials	Com. Date
❶	❷	❸	❹	❺	❻	❼

Document Database Preparation

Each circled number below corresponds to the circled number on the sample document database.

❶   Document Number: Enter the protocol, addendum, certification, deficiency or final report number.

Example: PV010-02.C01 (process validation protocol number)

❷   Description: Enter the document description.

Example: Balance, Precision, Mettler, Model AE10

❸   Equipment No.: Enter the equipment number, if applicable.

Example: 094

❹   Serial No: Enter the serial number, if applicable.

Example: P32739

❺   Location: Enter the location of equipment at the time of validation, if applicable.

❻   Initials: Enter the name of the person who produced the protocol.

❼   Com. Date: Enter the date when the document is complete.

*This is the first requal because the equipment was moved from the Dev Lab to the QC Lab.

℞	Document Database					
Document Number	**Description**	**Equip. No.**	**Serial No.**	**Location /Room**	**Name**	**Com. Date**
EV000-00	Balance, Precision, Mettler	0001	P32739	Dev Lab	PAC	09/24/97
EV000-00.A1	Balance, Precision, Mettler	0001	P32739	Dev Lab	PAC	09/10/97
EV000-00.C	Balance, Precision, Mettler	0001	P32739	Dev Lab	PAC	09/24/97
EV000-00.D1	Balance, Precision, Mettler	0001	P32739	Dev Lab	PAC	08/14/97
EV000-00.F	Balance, Precision, Mettler	0001	P32739	Dev Lab	PAC	09/25/97
EV000-01*	Balance, Precision, Mettler	0001	P32739	QC Lab	PAC	12/2/98
EV000-01.A1	etc.					
EV000-01.C						
EV000-01.F						
EV000-01						
EV000-02.A1						
EV000-02.C						
EV000-02.D1						
EV000-02.F						
Etc.						

Appendix A

Cleaning Qualification Protocol Example

I have included an actual qualification protocol template that is filled in to show you an example of how to develop a cleaning qualification protocol. Each of the protocol elements is covered in this template. This protocol covers the cleaning of just one piece of equipment, even though several pieces of equipment are used to process the product. Note that cleaning qualification protocols do not follow the usual IQ, OQ, and PQ format.

R̥	**Cleaning Qualification Protocol**	
Title: 800 Liter Vertical Mixer used to Manufacture (Product Name)		Protocol No.: 1009
Manufacturer: Any Mixer Co.		Page: 1 of 7
Model Number: AMP 800	Serial Number: 0932	
Equipment Number: 240	Location: Room 348	

Prepared By:		
Validation:		Date:
Approved By:		
Validation Manager:		Date:
Research & Development:		Date:
Operations:		Date:
Maintenance:		Date:
Regulatory Compliance:		Date:

R̽	**Cleaning Qualification Protocol**	
Protocol No.: 1009 Title: 800 Liter Vertical Mixer used to Manufacture (Product Name)		Page: 2 of 7

1.0 Table of Contents

Ŗ	**Cleaning Qualification Protocol**	
Protocol No.: 1009 Title: 800 Liter Vertical Mixer used to Manufacture (Product Name)		Page: 3 of 7

2.0 Objective

The objective of this cleaning qualification is to establish documented evidence that the 800 Liter mixer is acceptably cleaned and that the test results verified the effectiveness of the cleaning procedures used to remove product residue following the processing of (Product Name).

3.0 Scope

The scope of this cleaning qualification protocol includes the 800 Liter Mixer and its corresponding cleaning standard operating procedure.

4.0 Experimental

The manufacturing equipment under study will be sampled as detailed in analytical method GP CV-736, using Ethanol:Water 75/25% as the recovery solvent (based on solubility data for the active ingredients). A copy of the method is provided in Attachment 1. Method validation includes linearity, interference and recovery studies for representative product contact surface types.

The methodology includes an example standard chromatogram at $7.5\mu g$ and representative chromatogram of a solution at the limit of quantitation of $0.381 \mu g/mL$. Equipment minimum loads are determined from optimum operating ranges in the engineering standard that is on file in the Research and Development Department.

R	**Cleaning Qualification Protocol**	
Protocol No.: 1009 Title: 800 Liter Vertical Mixer used to Manufacture (Product Name)		Page: 4 of 7

4.1 Acceptance Criteria

A carry over of no more than 3 PPM of (Product Name) in a subsequent batch of material will be considered acceptable.

4.2 Sampling Plan

The walls, plow, chopper blade, discharge chute and lid of the 800 Liter Vertical Mixer will be rinsed with 75/25% v/v Ethanol/H_2O after the cleaning procedure and inspection. This procedure will apply for the validation of cleaning procedures after processing of (Product Name) formulations.

4.3 Test Procedure

Samples will be analyzed for residual levels of (Product Name) by Method VC-637. (See Attachment 1.) The following parameters will be determined before the analysis.

- Limit of detection and quantitation.

- Linearity over a given concentration range.

- Recovery of active material from representative product contact surfaces.

℞	**Cleaning Qualification Protocol**	
Protocol No.: 1009 Title: 800 Liter Vertical Mixer used to Manufacture (Product Name)		Page: 5 of 7

5.0 Validation Report

Following is the summary, experimental procedures, data and conclusions.

5.1 Test Results

The following Table I summarizes the test results for (Product Name) residuals for the piece of manufacturing equipment under test. The 800 Liter Vertical Mixer carryover is significantly lower than the 3 ppm limit specified.

Table I Cleaning Validation for (Product Name) 25 mg, Lot #02797

Equipment	Equipment No.	Next/Smallest Batch Size (g)	(Product Name) Total Amount Found (μg)	Residuals Amount Found (ppm)
800 Liter Vertical Mixer	240	150,000	311.62	0.0021

5.2 Summary

The cleaning validation test results verified the effectiveness of the cleaning procedures used to remove product residue following processing of (Product Name) in the 800 Liter Vertical Mixer.

Prepared By:	Date:
Verified By:	Date:

Ŗ	**Cleaning Qualification Protocol**	
Protocol No.: 1009 Title: 800 Liter Vertical Mixer used to Manufacture (Product Name)		Page: 6 of 7

Attachment 1

Analytical Methods for (Product Name)

℞	**Cleaning Qualification Protocol**	
Protocol No.: 1009 Title: 800 Liter Vertical Mixer used to Manufacture (Product Name)		Page: 7 of 7

Attachment 2

Batch Records

Appendix B

Facilities Qualification Protocol Example

I have included an actual qualification protocol template that is filled in to show you an example of how to develop a facilities qualification protocol. Each of the protocol elements is covered in the template.

R̥	**Facility Qualification Protocol**	
Title: Room 641 Enclosing Granulation Mixer		Protocol No.: 2047
Manufacturer: N/A		Page: 1 of 20
Model Number: N/A	Serial Number: N/A	
Equipment Number: N/A	Location: Room 641	
Prepared By:		
Validation:		Date:
Approved By:		
Validation Manager:		Date:
Research & Development:		Date:
Operations:		Date:
Maintenance:		Date:
Regulatory Compliance:		Date:

R̥	**Facility Qualification Protocol**	
Protocol No.: 2047 Title: Room 641 Enclosing Granulation Mixer		Page: 2 of 20

1.0   Table of Contents

℞	**Facility Qualification Protocol**	
Protocol No.: 2047 Title: Room 641 Enclosing Granulation Mixer		Page: 3 of 20

2.0   Objective

The objective of this facility qualification is to establish documented evidence that the Room 641 Enclosure is acceptably installed per manufacturer recommendations, process requirements, and/or engineering standards. Also the verification of: architectural drawings, dust collection, exhaust fan system, filter integrity test, HVAC critical components, SOPs, calibration of instruments in the room, microbial testing, light intensity testing, differential pressure testing, temperature and humidity control and differential pressure alarm activation.

3.0   Scope

The scope of this facility qualification protocol includes the Room 641 Enclosure and its associated components. Installation qualification is limited to the system components and includes installation of support utilities. Operational testing is limited to demonstrating component functionality.

4.0   Description

The Room 641 Enclosure was designed to enclose a granulation mixer. This enclosure will prevent cross contamination to and from other granulation rooms in operations. The enclosure is maintained at a negative pressure differential with respect to the surrounding area. The pressure differential is monitored and alarmed. All air introduced into the enclosure is filtered using HEPA filters at the point of entry into the enclosure. In order to maintain an adequate negative differential pressure, a booster fan is installed to remove air from the enclosure and deposit it into the staging area. The room is 9 feet by 16 feet.

5.0   Installation Qualification (IQ)

5.1   Required Documentation

5.1.1   Standard Operating Procedure

SOP# FAC045 Processing Room Checklist, Release Date: 04/17/98
SOP# FAC032 Processing Room Cleaning Procedure, Release Date: 09/12/98

℞	**Facility Qualification Protocol**	
Protocol No.: 2047 Title: Room 641 Enclosing Granulation Mixer		Page: 4 of 20

5.2 Architectural Verification Test

5.2.1 Test Objective

The objective of this verification is to ensure that the as-found conditions of the room comply with specifications. Information about utilities not specified by the manufacturer will be recorded as baseline information.

5.2.2 Test Procedure

Visually verify that all components specified on the as-built drawings match what is installed. Record the results in Table I. If there are any differences, red-line the facility drawings to show the differences.

Table I Architectural Verification Test Results

Feature	Specification	As-Found	Acceptable (Yes/No)
Room Dimensions	9' X 16' X 8'	As specified	Yes
Floor Material	Epoxy Terrazzo	As specified	Yes
Wall Material	PVC Sheets	As specified	Yes
Base Material	Epoxy Terrazzo	As specified	Yes
Ceiling Material	PVC Sheets	As specified	Yes
Lighting	Qty 2, 2' X 4'	As specified	Yes
Compressed Air Outlets	Qty 1	As specified	Yes
Breathable Air Outlets	Qty 1	As specified	Yes

Performed By:	Date:
Verified By:	Date:

℞	**Facility Qualification Protocol**	
Protocol No.: 2047 Title: Room 641 Enclosing Granulation Mixer		Page: 5 of 20

Table I Architectural Verification Test Results (Continued.)

Feature	Specification	As Found	Acceptable (Yes/No)
Potable Water Outlets	Qty 1	As specified	Yes
DC Inlets	Qty 2, Plenums	As specified	Yes
DC Supply	Qty 1, 2' X 4'	As specified	Yes
HVAC Supply Ducts	Qty 3, 2' X 4'	As specified	Yes
HEPA Filter	Qty 4, 2' X 4'	As specified	Yes
HVAC Return Ducts	Qty 1, 14" X 14"	As specified	Yes
Floor Drains	Qty 1	As specified	Yes
110 VDC Outlets	Qty 1	As specified	Yes
Equipment Electrical Connections	Qty 2	As specified	Yes
Fire Sprinklers	Qty 2	As specified	Yes

Performed By:	Date:
Verified By:	Date:

R	**Facility Qualification Protocol**	
Protocol No.: 2047 Title: Room 641 Enclosing Granulation Mixer		Page: 6 of 20

5.3   HVAC Components List

5.3.1   Test Objective

To document the pertinent information on the HVAC equipment.

5.3.2   Test Procedure

Record the information as indicated on the installed component in Table II.

Table II HVAC Components List Test Results

Component Name	AHU-3
Component Identification Tag Number	None
Manufacturer	Carrier
Model Number	026610RD84
Serial Number	2289G0944 Series DA

Performed By:	Date:
Verified By:	Date:

℞	**Facility Qualification Protocol**

Protocol No.: 2047 Title: Room 641 Enclosing Granulation Mixer	Page: 7 of 20

5.4   Dust Control Components List

5.4.1   Test Objective

To document the pertinent information on the Dust Control equipment.

5.4.2   Test Procedure

Record the information as indicated on the installed component in Table III.

Table III Dust Control Components List Test Results

Component Name	DC-33C
Component Identification Tag Number	862
Manufacturer	Torit
Model Number	055SV
Serial Number	778909

Performed By:	Date:
Verified By:	Date:

R̠	**Facility Qualification Protocol**	
Protocol No.: 2047 Title: Room 641 Enclosing Granulation Mixer		Page: 8 of 20

5.5   Exhaust Fan Components List

5.5.1   Test Objective

To document the pertinent information on the Exhaust Fan equipment.

5.5.2   Test Procedure

Record the information as indicated on the installed component in Table IV.

Table IV Exhaust Fan Components List Test Results

Component Name	EF-33 B
Component Identification Tag Number	649
Manufacturer	Cook
Model Number	100 CZB
Serial Number	54174

Performed By:		Date:
Verified By:		Date:

℞	**Facility Qualification Protocol**	
Protocol No.: 2047 Title: Room 641 Enclosing Granulation Mixer		Page: 9 of 20

5.6   Utilities Verification Test

5.6.1   Test Objective

To verify that the utilities are sufficient for the equipment used in the room.

5.6.2   Test Procedure

Record the information as indicated on the installed components in Table V and the instruments used to measure the volts and compressed air pressure in Table VI.

Table V Utilities Test Results

Utility	Specified	Measured Results	Acceptable (Yes/No)
Electrical	220 V AC	219 V AC	Yes
Compressed Air	80 psig	80 psig	Yes

Table VI   Instruments Used

Test Instrument	Identification No.	Cal Due Date
Multimeter	ME-025	04/19/98
Air Pressure Gauge	P-102	02/10/98

Performed By:	Date:
Verified By:	Date:

R	**Facility Qualification Protocol**	
Protocol No.: 2047 Title: Room 641 Enclosing Granulation Mixer		Page: 10 of 20

5.7   Calibration Requirements

5.7.1   Test Objective

This test verifies that all instruments have been evaluated for calibration requirements. It also verifies that the instruments requiring calibration have current calibration stickers, a calibration certificate and that the calibration is traceable to an NIST standard.

5.7.2   Test Procedure

Verify that all critical instruments are logged into the calibration system, have calibration procedures in place and are currently in calibration at the time of qualification testing. Record all of the necessary information for the calibrated instruments used with this room in Table VII and attach their certifications in Attachment 1.

Table VII Calibrated Instruments Test Results

Instrument	ID/Part Number	Cal Req'd (Yes/No)	Cal Due Date	Operating Range
Magnahelic Gauge	MFG HVAC DPG044	Yes	10/21/98	0 to 100 in. W.C.
Differential Pressure Gauge, Transmitter	MFG HVAC DPT045	Yes	10/25/98	-0.10 to + 0.10 in W.C.
Differential Pressure Gauge, Switch	MFG HVAC DPS046	Yes	10/21/98	0.4 to + 1.6 in W.C.

Performed By:		Date:
Verified By:		Date:

℞	**Facility Qualification Protocol**	
Protocol No.: 2047 Title: Room 641 Enclosing Granulation Mixer		Page: 11 of 20

6.0 Operational Qualification (OQ)

6.1 Microbial Test

6.1.1 Test Objective

Verify that the microbe count is acceptable for pharmaceutical manufacturing.

6.1.2 Test Procedure

Testing for airborne microbes is performed per PG M-8. Record the results in Table VIII.

Table VIII Microbial Test Results

Item	Results	Acceptable (Yes/No)
Total Plate Count	1 cfn/hr	Yes
Yeast and Mold Count	1 cfn/hr	Yes
Reference Document	3160 - 138	Yes

Performed By:		Date:
Verified By:		Date:

R̶	**Facility Qualification Protocol**	
Protocol No.: 2047 Title: Room 641 Enclosing Granulation Mixer		Page: 12 of 20

6.2 Light Intensity Test

6.2.1 Test Objective

Establish a baseline for the light intensity in the room.

6.2.2 Test Procedure

Measure the light intensity in the center of the room about 20" to 30" from the floor and record the results in Table IX.

Table IX Light Intensity Test Results

Item	Results	Acceptable (Yes/No)
Measured Light Intensity	33.6 Foot Candles	Yes

Performed By:	Date:
Verified By:	Date:

℞	**Facility Qualification Protocol**	
Protocol No.: 2047 Title: Room 641 Enclosing Granulation Mixer		Page: 13 of 20

6.3 HEPA Filter Integrity Test

6.3.1 Test Objective

The objective of this procedure is to verify the integrity of the HEPA filters and to verify that there were no leaks found during testing.

6.3.2 Test Procedure

Perform HEPA filter tests on all of the HEPA filters and record the results in Table X.

Table X HEPA Filter Integrity Test Results

Item	Specified	Results	Acceptable (Yes/No)
Filter No.	DC 215-1	As Specified	Yes
Filter Size	2' X 4'	As Specified	Yes
Photometer No.	21501	As Specified	Yes
Photometer Cal Date	N/S	10/6/98	Yes
Photometer Reading	< 0.01%	As Specified	Yes
Date of Test	N/S	01/15/98	Yes
Leaks	Yes/No	No	Yes

Performed By:		Date:
Verified By:		Date:

R̶	**Facility Qualification Protocol**	
Protocol No.: 2047 Title: Room 641 Enclosing Granulation Mixer		Page: 14 of 20

Table X HEPA Filter Integrity Test Results (Continued.)

Item	Specified	Results	Acceptable (Yes/No)
Filter No.	AC 215-1	As Specified	Yes
Filter Size	14" X 14"	As Specified	Yes
Photometer No.	21501	As Specified	Yes
Photometer Cal Date	N/S	10/6/98	Yes
Photometer Reading	< 0.01%	As Specified	Yes
Date of Test	N/S	01/15/98	Yes
Leaks	Yes/No	No	Yes
Filter No.	AC 215-2	As Specified	Yes
Filter Size	2' X 4'	As Specified	Yes
Photometer No.	21501	As Specified	Yes
Photometer Cal Date	N/S	10/6/98	Yes
Photometer Reading	< 0.01%	As Specified	Yes
Date of Test	N/S	01/15/98	Yes
Leaks	Yes/No	No	Yes

Performed By:	Date:
Verified By:	Date:

R	**Facility Qualification Protocol**		
Protocol No.: 2047 Title: Room 641 Enclosing Granulation Mixer			Page: 15 of 20

Table X HEPA Filter Integrity Test Results (Continued.)

Item	Specified	Results	Acceptable (Yes/No)
Filter No.	DC 215-3	As Specified	Yes
Filter Size	2' X 4'	As Specified	Yes
Photometer No.	21501	As Specified	Yes
Photometer Cal Date	N/S	10/6/98	Yes
Photometer Reading	< 0.01%	As Specified	Yes
Date of Test	N/S	01/15/98	Yes
Leaks	Yes/No	No	Yes
Filter No.	DC 215-4	As Specified	Yes
Filter Size	2' X 4'	As Specified	Yes
Photometer No.	21501	As Specified	Yes
Photometer Cal Date	N/S	10/6/98	Yes
Photometer Reading	< 0.01%	As Specified	Yes
Date of Test	N/S	01/15/98	Yes
Leaks	Yes/No	No	Yes

Performed By:	Date:
Verified By:	Date:

R̥	**Facility Qualification Protocol**	
Protocol No.: 2047 Title: Room 641 Enclosing Granulation Mixer		Page: 16 of 20

7.0 Performance Qualification (PQ)

7.1 Air Balance Verification Test

7.1.1 Test Objective

The objective of this test is to determine the number of air changes in the room and determine if the static pressure is negative or positive.

7.1.2 Test Procedure

Measure the air flow of all of the supply and return air ducts, record the results in Table XI, and then add them up. Record the instrument used to measure the air flow in Table XII. Calculate the number of air changes in the room.

Table XI Utilities Test Results

Duct	Supply/Return	Measured Results (cfm)	Acceptable (Yes/No)
DC 512-1	Supply	21	Yes
AC 512-1	Supply	53	Yes
AC 512-2	Supply	55	Yes
AC 512-3	Supply	52	Yes
AC 512-4	Supply	53	Yes
HVAC	Return	-310	Yes
Total		-76	

Performed By:		Date:
Verified By:		Date:

R̥	Facility Qualification Protocol

Protocol No.: 2047 Title: Room 641 Enclosing Granulation Mixer	Page: 17 of 20

Room Air Change Calculation

Return cfm/min. X 60 min./hr. X 1 Room/Volume = Number of Room Air Changes/hr.

Room Air Changes = -76/min. X 60 min./hr. X 1 Room/1,152 = 3.9/hr.

Table XII   Instruments Used

Test Instrument	Identification No.	Calibration Due Date
Annometer	AM-78342	05/30/98

Performed By:	Date:
Verified By:	Date:

R	**Facility Qualification Protocol**	
Protocol No.: 2047 Title: Room 641 Enclosing Granulation Mixer		Page: 18 of 20

7.2 Differential Pressure Verification Test

7.2.1 Test Objective

The objective of this test is to verify that the differential pressure of the room is greater than or equal to 0.02 in. W.C. (negative) and the alarm system is functioning properly.

7.2.2 Test Procedure

1. With the door closed, record the air pressure on the magnehelic gauge and the color of the alarm light in Table XIII.

2. Open the door and record the air pressure of the room when the alarm light changes from green tc red in Table XIII.

3. With the door remaining open, record the air pressure on the magnehelic gauge and the color of the alarm light in Table XIII.

4. Close the door and record the air pressure of the room when the alarm light changes from red to green in Table XIII.

Table XIII Differential Pressure Test Results

Test No.	Door Position	Alarm Light Color	Pressure (in. W.C.)	Acceptable (Yes/No)
1	Closed	Green	0.04	Yes
2	Open	Green to Red	0.03	Yes
3	Open	Red	0.005	Yes
4	Closed	Red to Green	0.05	Yes

Performed By:		Date:
Verified By:		Date:

℞	**Facility Qualification Protocol**	
Protocol No.: 2047 Title: Room 641 Enclosing Granulation Mixer		Page: 19 of 20

7.3 Temperature and Humidity Control Test

7.3.1 Test Objective

The objective of this test is to verify that the HVAC/Dust Control system can maintain the room temperature and relative humidity at 70°F ±5°F.

7.3.2 Test Procedure

Under normal operating conditions, measure the air temperature in the rooms served by the HVAC unit. Measure the temperature and humidity in each of the corners (4) and in the center of the room, about 4 feet above the floor. Record the results in Table XIV.

Table XIV Temperature and Humidity Control Test Results

Date	NE Corner	NW Corner	SE Corner	SW Corner	Center	Acceptable (Yes/No)
05/16/98	70°F	70°F	69°F	70°F	71°F	Yes

Performed By:		Date:
Verified By:		Date:

R̽	**Facility Qualification Protocol**	
Protocol No.: 2047 Title: Room 641 Enclosing Granulation Mixer		Page: 20 of 20

Attachment 1

Test Equipment Calibration Certificates

Appendix C

Utilities Qualification Protocol Example

I have included an actual qualification protocol template that is filled in to show you an example of how to develop a utilities qualification protocol. Each of the protocol elements is covered in the template.

Ŗ	**Utility Qualification Protocol**	
Title: Distilled Water System, Laboratory		Protocol No.: 3034
Manufacturer: Mueller Water Systems		Page: 1 of 29
Model Number: SV-52	Serial Number: 49A1	
Equipment Number: SV-2DIST	Location: Laboratory Building	

Prepared By:	
Validation:	Date:
Approved By:	
Validation Manager:	Date:
Research & Development:	Date:
Operations:	Date:
Maintenance:	Date:
Regulatory Compliance:	Date:

℞	**Utility Qualification Protocol**	Protocol No.: 3034
	Title: Distilled Water System, Laboratory	Page: 2 of 29

1.0 Table of Contents

R̥	**Utility Qualification Protocol**	Protocol No.: 3034
Title: Distilled Water System, Laboratory		Page: 3 of 29

2.0   Objective

The objective of this utility qualification is to establish documented evidence that the Laboratory Distilled Water system is acceptably installed per manufacturer recommendations, process requirements, and/or engineering standards. Acceptable installation includes suitable utility connections, components, and critical instruments in current calibration. Acceptable operation includes, as applicable, proper control and sequencing functions, recording and reporting functions, and safety and alarm features that meet process requirements and System specifications. Acceptable performance includes consistent operation within specified process parameters under simulated or actual operating conditions.

3.0   Scope

The scope of this utility qualification protocol includes the water system and its associated components. Installation qualification is limited to the system components and includes supporting utilities. Operational testing is limited to demonstrating system functionality.

4.0   Water System Description

The laboratory Distilled Water System produces and distributes USP purified water for use in laboratory analysis. The system consists of two vapor compression stills, a storage tank with internal ultraviolet (UV) lights, a distribution pump, an in-line UV light located downstream of the pump and a distribution loop with use-points throughout the laboratory.

The deionized water from the laboratory DI water system is filtered and softened before being supplied to the vapor compression stills. The stills vaporize the water and separate out the impurities before recondensing the stream into purified water, which is collected in a storage tank. The stills operate on call from the level sensor in the tank. Water from the storage tank is circulated through the loop by the distribution pump. An ultraviolet light is installed in the distribution line just downstream of the pump to inhibit microbial growth in the system. The distribution loop supplies water to the various laboratory use-points. the end of the loop is fed back into the storage tank to provide continuous circulation in the system. The storage tank is equipped with UV lights to inhibit microbial growth.

R **Utility Qualification Protocol**	Protocol No.: 3034
Title: Distilled Water System, Laboratory	Page: 4 of 29

5.0 Installation Qualification (IQ)

An IQ evaluation will establish confidence that the Distilled Water System is properly installed. The installation must meet the manufacturer's specified guidelines along with design changes at installation. Also, the supporting electrical utilities must meet all electrical codes. The information required for an IQ evaluation should be: system identification, required documentation, system utility requirements, major component specifications, component material, lubricants and System safety features.

5.1 Water System Identification

Record the water system identification numbers in Table I, along with the following information: System manufacturer, purchase order number, model number, serial number, company assigned System number, and the location of the System.

Writing Tip: The following information is found on the nameplate (placard) attached to the system and the system manufacturer's installation and operations manual.

Table I   Water System Identification

Required Information	As-found Conditions
Manufacturer	Any Distilled Water System Co.
Purchase Order Number	023910
Model Number	SV-52
Serial Number	49A1
Water System Number	SV-2DIST
Location	Laboratory Building
Performed By:	Date:
Verified By:	Date:

R̶ **Utility Qualification Protocol**	Protocol No.: 3034
Title: Distilled Water System, Laboratory	Page: 5 of 29

5.2   Required Documentation

Record the manufacturer's operation and maintenance manual and drawings in Table II.
Record the standard operating procedures that cover the setup, operation and cleaning of
the water system in Table III.

Table II   Required Documentation

Number	Description	Date
9202	Installation and Operation Instructions	5/96
None	Ultraviolet Water Purifiers	None

Table III   Standard Operating Procedures

Number	Description	Release Date
LAB036	Laboratory Purified Water System for Production USP Purified Water	07/30/95
LAB038	Purified Water Testing	03/25/95

5.3   Water System Utility Requirements

Compare the manufacturer's specified volt (V) and amps (A), and water pressure
requirements to their as-found condition at the time of qualification testing and record the
results in Table IV. Also, record the location of the power supply source. Record the
instrument used to measure the volts, amps and water pressure in Table V.

Performed By:	Date:
Verified By:	Date:

R̥	**Utility Qualification Protocol**	Protocol No.: 3034

Title: Distilled Water System, Laboratory	Page: 6 of 29

Volt Calculation:

Volt specification = 220 V ±10%
±10% of 220 = ±22
220 + 22 = 242
220 - 22 = 198
The measured volts of 221/220/223 fall within ±10%.

Amp Calculation:

Circuit rating = 20 A
System current draw = 15 A
The circuit amp rating of 20 is greater than the maximum current draw of the System.

Water Pressure Calculation:

Supply DI Water specification ≥ 40 psig
The measured water pressure of 59 psig is greater than 40 psig.

Table IV   Utilities

Utility	Specified	Measured Results	Acceptable (Yes/No)
Volts	220 ±10%	A-B 221 A-C 220 B-C 223	Yes
Amps	Pump = 15	20 Circuit Rating	Yes
Water	Pressure ≥ 40 psig	59 psig	Yes

Power supply source, breaker box BB29, wire numbers: 17, 19, 21.

Performed By:	Date:
Verified By:	Date:

℞	**Utility Qualification Protocol**	Protocol No.: 3034
Title: Distilled Water System, Laboratory		Page: 7 of 29

Table V   Instrument Used

Test Instrument	**Identification Number**	**Calibration Due Date**
Multimeter	ME-025	04/19/97
Water Pressure Gauge	PA-102	10/13/96

5.4   Major Component Specifications

This section is used to verify that the water system components purchased were delivered and installed. Record the major components in Table VI.

Table VI   Major Components

#	**Components**	**As-found**	**Leaks (Yes/No)**
1	Shut Off Valve	Spears 1/2" PVC	No
2	Check Valve	TVI 3/4" PVC	No
3	Sample Port	1/4" PVC	No
4	Shut Off Valve	TVI 3/4" PVC	No
5	Shut Off Valve	TVI 3/4" PVC	No
6	Hardness Monitor	Mueller	No
7	Water Softener	Not specified.	No
8	Shut Off Valve	TVI 3/4" PVC	No
9	Pressure Switch	Furnas	No
Performed By:			Date:
Verified By:			Date:

Ŗ	Utility Qualification Protocol		Protocol No.: 3034
Title: Distilled Water System, Laboratory			Page: 8 of 29

Table VI Major Components (Continued.)

#	Components	As-found	Leaks (Yes/No)
10	Pressure Pump	Manufacturer: Teel Model number: 51CE2H84C Serial number: 49A1 hp: 1/2	No
11	Pressure Tank	Manufacturer: Teel Model number: 438P4	No
12	Check Valve	TVI 3/4" PVC	No
13	Relief Valve	Press - 75	No
14	Conductivity Probe	Type: 112-1 Serial number: 93136	No
15	Shut Off Valve	TVI 3/4" PVC	No
16	Shut Off Valve	TVI 3/4" PVC	No
17	1μ Filter	Not specified.	No
18	Shut Off Valve	TVI 3/4" PVC	No
19	Sample Port	Manufacturer: Nibco	No
20	Pressure Regulator	Manufacturer: Watts Model number: 3AG24-05 Serial number: 4229 Thread Size: 1/2" NPT	No
21	Pressure Gauge	Manufacturer: Noshok Range: 0 - 100 psig	No

Performed By:	Date:
Verified By:	Date:

R	Utility Qualification Protocol	Protocol No.: 3034
Title: Distilled Water System, Laboratory		Page: 9 of 29

Table VI   Major Components (Continued.)

#	Components	As-found	Leaks (Yes/No)
22	Pressure Switch	Manufacturer: Furnas	No
23	Shut Off Valve	Spears 1/2" PVC	No
24	Still No. 1	Manufacturer: Muller Model number: 5356088 Serial number: AC8202	No
25	Shut Off Valve	Spears 1/2" PVC	No
26	Shut Off Valve	Spears 1/2" PVC	No
27	Still No. 2	Manufacturer: Muller Model number: 5356088 Serial number: AC8203	No
28	Shut Off Valve	Spears 1/2" PVC	No
29	Overfill Protection	Not specified.	No
30	Water Tank	Manufacturer: Muller Part number: 167905 Serial number: 928331	No
31	Shut Off Valve	Spears 3/4" PVC	No
32	Shut Off Valve	Manufacturer: Teel Thread size: 1/2" NPT	No
33	Pump	Manufacturer: Price Pump Co. Model number: 161B Serial number: 35-11LB hp: 1/2	No

Performed By:	Date:
Verified By:	Date:

| R̥ | **Utility Qualification Protocol** | Protocol No.: 3034 |

| Title: Distilled Water System, Laboratory | Page: 10 of 29 |

Table VI Major Components (Continued.)

#	Components	As-found	Leaks (Yes/No)
34	Shut Off Valve	TVI 3/4" PVC	No
35	Shut Off Valve	TVI 3/4" PVC	No
36	UV Light	Manufacturer: Ultra Dyn Part number: FB-0051 Serial number: W53549	No
37	Shut Off Valve	TVI 3/4" PVC	No
38	Shut Off Valve	TVI 1" PVC	No
39	Shut Off Valve	TVI 1/2" PVC	No
40	Shut Off Valve	TVI 1" PVC	No
1A	Faucet	Manufacturer: Spears Material: PVC	No
1B	Faucet	Manufacturer: Spears Material: PVC	No
2A	Faucet	Manufacturer: Spears Material: PVC	No
2B	Faucet	Manufacturer: Spears Material: PVC	No
3A	Faucet	Manufacturer: Spears Material: PVC	No

| Performed By: | Date: |
| Verified By: | Date: |

Ŗ	**Utility Qualification Protocol**		Protocol No.: 3034

Title: Distilled Water System, Laboratory		Page: 11 of 29

Table VI   Major Components (Continued.)

#	Components	As-found	Leaks (Yes/No)
3B	Faucet	Manufacturer: Spears Material: PVC	No
3C	Faucet	Manufacturer: Spears Material: PVC	No
3D	Faucet	Manufacturer: Spears Material: PVC	No
4A	Faucet	Manufacturer: Spears Material: PVC	No
4B	Faucet	Manufacturer: Spears Material: PVC	No
5A	Faucet	Manufacturer: Spears Material: PVC	No
5B	Faucet	Manufacturer: Spears Material: PVC	No
5C	Faucet	Manufacturer: Spears Material: PVC	No
5D	Faucet	Manufacturer: Spears Material: PVC	No
6A	Faucet	Manufacturer: Spears Material: PVC	No

Performed By:	Date:
Verified By:	Date:

R	**Utility Qualification Protocol**		Protocol No.: 3034
Title: Distilled Water System, Laboratory			Page: 12 of 29

Table VI Major Components (Continued.)

#	Components	As-found	Leaks (Yes/No)
6B	Faucet	Manufacturer: Spears Material: PVC	No
7A	Faucet	Manufacturer: Spears Material: PVC	No
7B	Faucet	Manufacturer: Spears Material: PVC	No
7C	Faucet	Manufacturer: Spears Material: PVC	No
7D	Faucet	Manufacturer: Spears Material: PVC	No
8A	Faucet	Manufacturer: Spears Material: PVC	No
8B	Faucet	Manufacturer: Spears Material: PVC	No
9A	Faucet	Manufacturer: Spears Material: PVC	No
9B	Faucet	Manufacturer: Spears Material: PVC	No
10A	Faucet	Manufacturer: Spears Material: PVC	No

Performed By:	Date:
Verified By:	Date:

R	**Utility Qualification Protocol**	Protocol No.: 3034

Title: Distilled Water System, Laboratory	Page: 13 of 29

Table VI   Major Components (Continued.)

#	Components	As-found	Leaks (Yes/No)
10B	Faucet	Manufacturer: Spears Material: PVC	No
11A	Faucet	Manufacturer: Spears Material: PVC	No
11B	Faucet	Manufacturer: Spears Material: PVC	No
11C	Faucet	Manufacturer: Spears Material: PVC	No
11D	Faucet	Manufacturer: Spears Material: PVC	No
12A	Faucet	Manufacturer: Spears Material: PVC	No
12B	Faucet	Manufacturer: Spears Material: PVC	No
13A	Faucet	Manufacturer: Spears Material: PVC	No
13B	Faucet	Manufacturer: Spears Material: PVC	No
13C	Faucet	Manufacturer: Spears Material: PVC	No

Performed By:	Date:
Verified By:	Date:

R **Utility Qualification Protocol**		Protocol No.: 3034
Title: Distilled Water System, Laboratory		Page: 14 of 29

Table VI   Major Components (Continued.)

#	Components	As-found	Leaks (Yes/No)
13D	Faucet	Manufacturer: Spears Material: PVC	No
14A	Faucet	Manufacturer: Spears Material: PVC	No
14B	Faucet	Manufacturer: Spears Material: PVC	No
15A	Faucet	Manufacturer: Spears Material: PVC	No
15B	Faucet	Manufacturer: Spears Material: PVC	No
15C	Faucet	Manufacturer: Spears Material: PVC	No
15D	Faucet	Manufacturer: Spears Material: PVC	No
16A	Faucet	Manufacturer: Spears Material: PVC	No
16B	Faucet	Manufacturer: Spears Material: PVC	No
17A	Faucet	Manufacturer: Spears Material: PVC	No

Performed By:	Date:
Verified By:	Date:

℞	**Utility Qualification Protocol**		Protocol No.: 3034
Title: Distilled Water System, Laboratory			Page: 15 of 29

Table VI   Major Components (Continued.)

#	Components	As-found	Leaks (Yes/No)
17B	Faucet	Manufacturer: Spears Material: PVC	No
17C	Faucet	Manufacturer: Spears Material: PVC	No
17D	Faucet	Manufacturer: Spears Material: PVC	No
18A	Faucet	Manufacturer: Spears Material: PVC	No
18B	Faucet	Manufacturer: Spears Material: PVC	No
19A	Faucet	Manufacturer: Spears Material: PVC	No
19B	Faucet	Manufacturer: Spears Material: PVC	No
19C	Faucet	Manufacturer: Spears Material: PVC	No
19D	Faucet	Manufacturer: Spears Material: PVC	No
20A	Faucet	Manufacturer: Spears Material: PVC	No

Performed By:	Date:
Verified By:	Date:

R	**Utility Qualification Protocol**	Protocol No.: 3034
Title: Distilled Water System, Laboratory		Page: 16 of 29

Table VI Major Components (Continued.)

#	Components	As-found	Leaks (Yes/No)
20B	Faucet	Manufacturer: Spears Material: PVC	No
21A	Faucet	Manufacturer: Spears Material: PVC	No
21B	Faucet	Manufacturer: Spears Material: PVC	No
22A	Faucet	Manufacturer: Spears Material: PVC	No
23A	Faucet	Manufacturer: Spears Material: PVC	No
23B	Faucet	Manufacturer: Spears Material: PVC	No
24A	Faucet	Manufacturer: Spears Material: PVC	No
24B	Faucet	Manufacturer: Spears Material: PVC	No
24C	Faucet	Manufacturer: Spears Material: PVC	No
25A	Faucet	Manufacturer: Spears Material: PVC	No

Performed By:	Date:
Verified By:	Date:

R	Utility Qualification Protocol		Protocol No.: 3034

Title: Distilled Water System, Laboratory	Page: 17 of 29

Table VI   Major Components (Continued.)

#	Components	As-found	Leaks (Yes/No)
26A	Faucet	Manufacturer: Spears Material: PVC	No
27B	Faucet	Manufacturer: Spears Material: PVC	No
28	Faucet	Manufacturer: Spears Material: PVC	No
NE Wall	Shut Off Valve	TVI 1/2" PVC	No
North	Shut Off Valve	TVI 1/2" PVC	No
Mid	Shut Off Valve	TVI 1/2" PVC	No
South	Shut Off Valve	TVI 1/2" PVC	No
NC	Shut Off Valve	Spears 1/2" PVC	No
SC	Shut Off Valve	Spears 1/2" PVC	No
29	Faucet	Manufacturer: Spears Material: PVC	No
30	Faucet	Manufacturer: Spears Material: PVC	No
31	Faucet	Manufacturer: Spears Material: PVC	No
32	Faucet	Manufacturer: Spears Material: PVC	No
Performed By:			Date:
Verified By:			Date:

R̥ **Utility Qualification Protocol**	Protocol No.: 3034
Title: Distilled Water System, Laboratory	Page: 18 of 29

5.5 Component Material

Record the material of each component that contacts the product in Table VII.

Table VII Component Material

Component	Material
None.	

5.6 Lubricants

Record the lubricant used to operate the water system in Table VIII and indicate if they make contact with the product. Is there is a preventive maintenance procedure on file? (Yes/No) Yes

Table VIII Lubricants

Where Used	Type	Manufacturer	Product Contact (Yes/No)
None.			

5.7 Water System Safety Features

Test Objective. The objective of this test is to verify that the safety features for the water system function according to the manufacturer's specifications.

Test Procedure.

- Verify that all of the safety features are operational and record the results in Table IX .

Performed By:	Date:
Verified By:	Date:

R̠	**Utility Qualification Protocol**	Protocol No.: 3034
Title: Distilled Water System, Laboratory		Page: 19 of 29

Table IX   Safety Features Test Results

Test Function	Expected Results	Acceptable (Yes/No)
Interlock Switch	The still shuts off when placed in the regeneration mode.	Yes
Low Pressure Switch	The supply water shuts off when the water pressure drops below 40 psig.	Yes
Conductivity Probe	The still shuts off when the resistance on conductivity meter drops below the preset reading.	Yes
Magnetic Switch No. 1	The still shuts off when the tank is full.	Yes
Magnetic Switch No. 2	The still #2 is activated when the water level drops below the magnetic switch.	Yes

6.0   Operational Qualification (OQ)

An OQ evaluation should establish that the water system can operate within specified tolerances and limits. The information required for the OQ evaluation should be: calibration of the instrument used to control the water system, control functions (switches and pushbuttons) and system operation.

6.1   Calibration Requirements

Verify that all critical instruments for the water system are logged into the calibration system, have calibration procedures in place and are currently in calibration at the time of qualification testing. Record all of the necessary information for the calibrated instruments used to control the water system in Table X.

Performed By:	Date:
Verified By:	Date:

R	**Utility Qualification Protocol**	Protocol No.: 3034
	Title: Distilled Water System, Laboratory	Page: 20 of 29

Table X Calibrated Instruments

Instrument	As-found Conditions
Identification number	100-GP
Type	Water pressure gauge, analog
Manufacturer	Any Gauge Co.
Model number	8441J
Serial number	F1
Range	0 to 100 psig
Scale division	2 psig
Location	On instrument panel.
Use	Monitors the DI water pressure.
Calibration due date	07/08/97
Critical or not critical	Critical

Prepared By:	Date:
Verified By:	Date:

R̶ **Utility Qualification Protocol**	Protocol No.: 3034
Title: Distilled Water System, Laboratory	Page: 21 of 29

Table X   Calibrated Instruments (Continued.)

Instrument	As-found Conditions
Identification number	200-GP
Type	Water pressure gauge, analog
Manufacturer	Any Gauge Co.
Model number	8441J
Serial number	F2
Range	0 to 100 psig
Scale division	2 psig
Location	On instrument panel.
Use	Monitors the DI water pressure.
Calibration due date	07/08/97
Critical or not critical	Critical

Prepared By:	Date:
Verified By:	Date:

R **Utility Qualification Protocol**		Protocol No.: 3034
Title: Distilled Water System, Laboratory		Page: 22 of 29

Table X   Calibrated Instruments (Continued.)

Instrument	As-found Conditions
Identification number	300-GP
Type	Water pressure gauge, analog
Manufacturer	Any Gauge Co.
Model number	8441J
Serial number	F3
Range	0 to 100 psig
Scale division	2 psig
Location	On instrument panel.
Use	Monitors the DI water pressure.
Calibration due date	07/08/97
Critical or not critical	Critical

Prepared By:	Date:
Verified By:	Date:

℞	**Utility Qualification Protocol**	Protocol No.: 3034
Title: Distilled Water System, Laboratory		Page: 23 of 29

7.0   Performance Qualification (PQ)

Once it has been established that the water system is properly installed and functioning within specified operating parameters, it must be shown that the water system can be operated reliably under routine operating conditions.

7.1   USP Quality Standards for Purified Water Acceptance Criteria

Chemical Content	Method	Limit
pH	USP XXII pg. 1457	5.0 to 7.0
Chloride	USP XXII pg. 1457	No opalescence produced
Sulfate	USP XXII pg. 1457	No turbidity
Ammonia	USP XXII pg. 1457	Not darker than control
Calcium	USP XXII pg. 1457	No turbidity
Carbon Dioxide	USP XXII pg. 1457	Mixture remains clear
Heavy Metals	USP XXII pg. 1457	Not darker than standard
Oxidizables	USP XXII pg. 1457	Pink does not disappear
Total Solids	USP XXII pg. 1457	NMT 1 mg of residue
Bacteria (Total Colony Count)	Company Standard	NMT 100 cfu/ml
Coliforms	Company Standard	NMT 0 cfu/ml
Pseudomonas Species	Company Standard	NMT 0 cfu/ml

Prepared By:	Date:
Verified By:	Date:

Ŗ **Utility Qualification Protocol**	Protocol No.: 3034
Title: Distilled Water System, Laboratory	Page: 24 of 29

7.2 Chemical Test Procedure

Remove Distilled Water samples for 30 consecutive days. The samples will be taken from 6 distilled use points on the South wall, Northwest wall, Robotics room North, middle and South sites and 72 bench site faucets throughout the laboratory. Three bench site faucets, 3 wall units and 3 robotics units per day will be rotated through the 30 day period. Prior to sampling, a 25 second flush will need to be performed. This is based on 1/2" pipe diameter. A conversion factor of 0.016 X the longest deadleg section of approximately 40 feet to a 25 second flush. Record the results in Attachment 2.

7.3 Microbiological Test Procedure

Microbiological testing will be performed on each sample, except the point of use samples. Perform microbial testing for 30 days in accordance with Company Standard, Method M-1 Water Analysis. Record the results in Attachment 3.

℞ **Utility Qualification Protocol**	Protocol No.: 3034
Title: Distilled Water System, Laboratory	Page: 25 of 29

Attachment 1

Calibration Certifications

R	**Utility Qualification Protocol**	Protocol No.: 3034
Title: Distilled Water System, Laboratory		Page: 26 of 29

Attachment 2

Chemical Test Results

Sample Date	Chloride *	Sulfate *	Ammonia *	Calcium *	Carbon Dioxide *	Heavy Metal *	Oxidizable *	Total Solids *
10/22/97	Yes	Yes	Yes	Yes	Yes	Yes	Yes	Yes
10/23/97	Yes	Yes	Yes	Yes	Yes	Yes	Yes	Yes
10/24/97	Yes	Yes	Yes	Yes	Yes	Yes	Yes	Yes
10/25/97	Yes	Yes	Yes	Yes	Yes	Yes	Yes	Yes
10/26/97	Yes	Yes	Yes	Yes	Yes	Yes	Yes	Yes
10/27/97	Yes	Yes	Yes	Yes	Yes	Yes	Yes	Yes
10/28/97	Yes	Yes	Yes	Yes	Yes	Yes	Yes	Yes
10/29/97	Yes	Yes	Yes	Yes	Yes	Yes	Yes	Yes
10/30/97	Yes	Yes	Yes	Yes	Yes	Yes	Yes	Yes
10/31/97	Yes	Yes	Yes	Yes	Yes	Yes	Yes	Yes
11/1/97	Yes	Yes	Yes	Yes	Yes	Yes	Yes	Yes
11/2/97	Yes	Yes	Yes	Yes	Yes	Yes	Yes	Yes
11/3/97	Yes	Yes	Yes	Yes	Yes	Yes	Yes	Yes
11/4/97	Yes	Yes	Yes	Yes	Yes	Yes	Yes	Yes
11/5/97	Yes	Yes	Yes	Yes	Yes	Yes	Yes	Yes
11/6/97	Yes	Yes	Yes	Yes	Yes	Yes	Yes	Yes

* Meets specification? (Yes/No)

Ŗ̌	**Utility Qualification Protocol**	Protocol No.: 3034

Title: Distilled Water System, Laboratory	Page: 27 of 29

Attachment 2

Chemical Test Results (Continued.)

Sample Date	Chloride *	Sulfate *	Ammonia *	Calcium *	Carbon Dioxide *	Heavy Metal *	Oxidizable *	Total Solids *
11/7/97	Yes	Yes	Yes	Yes	Yes	Yes	Yes	Yes
11/8/97	Yes	Yes	Yes	Yes	Yes	Yes	Yes	Yes
11/9/97	Yes	Yes	Yes	Yes	Yes	Yes	Yes	Yes
11/10/97	Yes	Yes	Yes	Yes	Yes	Yes	Yes	Yes
11/11/97	Yes	Yes	Yes	Yes	Yes	Yes	Yes	Yes
11/12/97	Yes	Yes	Yes	Yes	Yes	Yes	Yes	Yes
11/13/97	Yes	Yes	Yes	Yes	Yes	Yes	Yes	Yes
11/14/97	Yes	Yes	Yes	Yes	Yes	Yes	Yes	Yes
11/15/97	Yes	Yes	Yes	Yes	Yes	Yes	Yes	Yes
11/16/97	Yes	Yes	Yes	Yes	Yes	Yes	Yes	Yes
11/17/97	Yes	Yes	Yes	Yes	Yes	Yes	Yes	Yes
11/18/97	Yes	Yes	Yes	Yes	Yes	Yes	Yes	Yes
11/19/97	Yes	Yes	Yes	Yes	Yes	Yes	Yes	Yes
11/20/97	Yes	Yes	Yes	Yes	Yes	Yes	Yes	Yes

* Meets specification? (Yes/No)

R	**Utility Qualification Protocol**	Protocol No.: 3034
	Title: Distilled Water System, Laboratory	Page: 28 of 29

Attachment 3

Microbial Test Results

Sample Date	Wall Site	TPC	Robot Site	TPC	Faucet Site	TPC	Faucet Site	TPC	Faucet Site	TPC
10/22/97	NW	10	N	23	1 A	1	11 C	11	24 B	6
10/23/97	NE	3064	M	125	1 A	5	13 B	1	21 B	5
10/24/97	S	30	M	55	1 A	4	7 B	11	17 D	1
10/25/97	NW	14	S	13	1 A	44	15 D	3	23 B	1
10/26/97	NE	6	N	1150	1 A	2	9 B	3	28 B	4
10/27/97	S	185	M	135	1 A	11	7 A	25	16 B	11
10/28/97	NW	1549	S	14	1 A	10	3 D	130	15 C	75
10/29/97	NE	75	N	235	1 A	2	5 D	5	11 D	55
10/30/97	S	172	M	27	1 A	1	5 B	13	19 C	29
10/31/97	NW	13	S	53	1 A	5	13 D	20	17 B	21
11/1/97	NE	155	N	165	1 A	2	7 C	38	30	140
11/2/97	S	7	M	850	1 A	4	26 A	142	31	29
11/3/97	NW	27	S	115	1 A	2	14 A	33	29	135
11/4/97	NE	60	N	350	1 A	5	12 B	40	28	77
11/5/97	S	39	M	225	1 A	3	8 A	49	22 A	210
11/6/97	NW	19	S	215	1 A	2	2 A	50	25 B	55
11/7/97	NE	65	N	1036	1 A	1	11 B	21	27	41
11/8/97	S	17	M	191	1 A	1	8 C	15	20 A	71
11/9/97	NW	47	S	127	1 A	1	4 A	53	6 A	23
11/10/97	NE	64	N	235	1 A	1	10 A	34	24 A	35
11/11/97	S	23	M	1045	1 A	2	19 A	175	19 B	120
11/12/97	NW	49	S	42	1 A	4	3 B	100	14 B	75

R̥ **Utility Qualification Protocol**								Protocol No.: 3034	
Title: Distilled Water System, Laboratory								Page: 29 of 29	

Attachment 3

Microbial Test Results (Continued.)

Sample Date	Wall Site	TPC	Robot Site	TPC	Faucet Site	TPC	Faucet Site	TPC	Faucet Site	TPC
11/13/97	NE	60	M	1045	1 A	1	12 A	17	21 A	26
11/14/97	S	597	S	200	1 A	1	11 B	1	16 A	14
11/15/97	NW	10	N	34	1 A	1	1 B	9	20 B	23
11/16/97	NE	40	M	52	1 A	2	5 A	24	17 A	34
11/17/97	S	8	S	220	1 A	1	10 B	24	13 A	38
11/18/97	NW	67	N	70	1 A	13	6 B	7	15 A	50
11/19/97	NE	1	M	12	1 A	1	2 CB	7	18 A	20
11/20/97	S	157	S	15	1 A	3	3 A	4	19 D	20

Appendix D

Equipment Qualification
Protocol Example

Figure D.1 is an actual qualification protocol template, filled in to show you how to develop a protocol. Each of the protocol elements is covered in the template: certification, final report, protocol, deficiency, and addendum.

See Chapter 8 under "Protocol Package Contents Sheet" for information on how to develop and use a protocol package contents sheet.

Figure D.1   **Protocol Documentation**

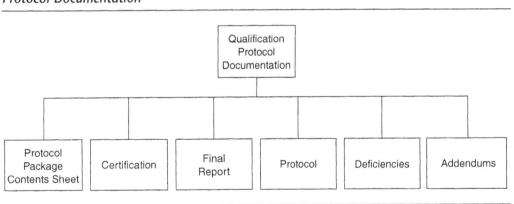

℞	Protocol Package Contents Sheet		
Equipment Name: (Any Mixer Co.) Model ME501 Emulsifying Mixer			
Equipment No.: *4010* Model No.: *MC501* Serial No.: *55356 B*		**Included:**	
Number	**Description**	**Yes**	**No**
CF001	Certification, Equipment	✔	
FR001	Final Report	✔	
4010	Protocol	✔	
	Capitol App. Request		✔
	Quote		✔
	Purchase Requisition		✔
0121577	Purchase Order	✔	
8110	Invoice	✔	
	Packing Slip		✔
No number	Vendor Spec Sheet	✔	
No number	Vendor Catalog: Emulsifying Mixer	✔	
No number	Equipment Manual: Installation and Operation	✔	
00862 00871	Main Drive Drawing Control System Drawing	✔	
GRA025	SOP: Granulation Equipment Setup	✔	
No number	Engineering Standard	✔	
No number	Preventive Maint Schedule: Monthly and 6 months	✔	
MTE-012	Calibration Certificates- Equipment Critical Instruments: MTE-FACILITIES	✔	
ME-025	Calibration Certificates-Test Instrument Multimeter	✔	

Form Number: V008 (5/28/98)   Reference: SOP-VAL008

See Chapter 5 under "System Certification" for information on how to develop and use a certification form.

℞	**Certification Form**	
Protocol No.: 4010 Title: (Any Mixer Co.) Model ME501 Emulsifying Mixer		CF No.: 001
Manufacturer: Any Mixer Co.		
Model Number: MC501	Serial Number: 55356 B	
Equipment Number: 2052	Location: Room 802 (This equipment is portable.)	

Statement

Based upon the acceptable results of the qualification testing and any applicable follow-up actions, this **Model ME501 Emulsifying Mixer** has been found to meet all validation requirements defined herein.

Originator:	Date:
Approved By: Manager of Validation:	Date:
Originator:	Date:
Approved By: Manager of Validation:	Date:
Originator:	Date:
Approved By: Manager of Validation:	Date:

Form Number: V004 (5/28/98)   Reference: SOP-VAL004

See Chapter 5 under "Final Report" for information on how to develop and use a final report.

℞	**Final Report**	
Protocol No.: 4056 Title: (Any Encapsulator Co.) Model GM200 Capsule Filler		FR No.: 001
Manufacturer: Any Encapsulator Co.		Page: 1 of 2
Model Number: GM200	Serial Number: Y67291	
Equipment Number: 371	Location: Room 539	

Abstract

The encapsulator is a new piece of equipment that is made up of several major components. It is controlled by a programmable logic controller (PLC). On the powder dosing unit the powder chamber, compression and layer values are modified by drives that are integrated in the machine logic and controlled by the PLC. The pellet dosing unit is entirely integrated in the machine logic and handled by the PLC.

The software program was evaluated against the functional requirements and the intended use of the equipment. The EEPROM was removed from the machine by the vendor so they could make changes at their home office. The program that was on the EEPROM was loaded into the RAM of the PLC so that the machine could be operated. The new software upgrade was received and installed. See Addendum A023, against protocol 4056.

Prepared By:	
Validation:	Date:
Approved By:	
Validation Manager:	Date:
Research & Development:	Date:
Operations:	Date:
Maintenance:	Date:
Regulatory Compliance:	Date:

R	Final Report	
Protocol No.: 4650		FR No.: 001
Title: (Any Encapsulator Co.) Model GM200 Capsule Filler		Page: 2 of 2

Installation Qualification

The unit was installed properly and all components were present. All applicable procedures were in place. The utilities supplied to the unit were inspected and found to be acceptable for proper operation of the unit.

Operational Qualification

All control and operational test function results were acceptable per the protocol test requirements. All alarms and safety devices functioned acceptably per the protocol test requirements except for the door interlocks that did not operate properly. See attached deficiency D075 against protocol 4056.

Performance Qualification

All performance testing was acceptable per the protocol test requirements. The following item was a deviation from the original qualification protocol.

Dev.#	Deviation	Protocol Page(s)
1	The original speed was measured with a hand held tachometer. This information was lined out and initialed and dated and a new measurement was taken with a calibrated remote speed controller that was specifically manufactured for this equipment.	21

Conclusion

The capsule filler has been tested and verified to operate properly according to manufacturer and process specifications. All corrections were noted in the protocol and a deficiency and an addendum were required.

See Chapter 3 under "Protocol Format" for information on how to develop and use a protocol.

℞	**Equipment Qualification Protocol**	
Title: (Any Mixer Co.) Model ME501 Emulsifying Mixer		Protocol No.: 4010
Manufacturer: Any Mixer Co.		Page: 1 of 21
Model Number: MC501	Serial Number: 55356 B	
Equipment Number: 2052	Location: Room 802 (This equipment is portable.)	
	Prepared By:	
Validation:		Date:
	Approved By:	
Validation Manager:		Date:
Research & Development:		Date:
Operations:		Date:
Maintenance:		Date:
Regulatory Compliance:		Date:

R̂ **Equipment Qualification Protocol**	Protocol No.: 4010
Title: (Any Mixer Co.) Model ME501 Emulsifying Mixer	Page: 2 of 21

Table of Contents

℞ **Equipment Qualification Protocol**	Protocol No.: 4010
Title: (Any Mixer Co.) Model ME501 Emulsifying Mixer	Page: 3 of 21

2.0 Objective

The objective of this equipment qualification is to establish documented evidence that the emulsifying mixer is acceptably installed per manufacturer recommendations, process requirements, and/or engineering standards. Acceptable installation includes suitable utility connections, components, and critical instruments in current calibration. Is fully operational as specified by the protocol. Acceptable operation includes, as applicable, proper control and sequencing functions, recording and reporting functions, and safety and alarm features that meet process requirements and equipment specifications. Acceptable performance includes consistent operation within specified process parameters under simulated or actual production conditions.

3.0 Scope

The scope of this equipment qualification protocol includes the emulsifying mixer and its associated components. Installation qualification is limited to the system components and does not include installation of support utilities, other than the connections at the system boundary. Operational testing is limited to demonstrating equipment functionality. Product specific testing is outside the scope of this qualification document, other than where a product is used to demonstrate equipment functionality.

4.0   Equipment Description

This section will explain how to validate an emulsifying mixer that is motor driven and operates at a fixed speed. All mixing operations are operator controlled with respect to duration and endpoint determination. The mixer provides high shear agitation to moderately low viscosity fluids. As viscosity and/or density increase the volume that the mixer will be able to handle effectively will decrease. The mixer is used in the preparation of solutions for use in a wet granulation process. The mixer cannot be operated without the impeller being submerged in water or other representative fluid or powder.

℞ Equipment Qualification Protocol	Protocol No.: 4010
Title: (Any Mixer Co.) Model ME501 Emulsifying Mixer	Page: 4 of 21

5.0 Installation Qualification (IQ)

An IQ evaluation will establish confidence that the equipment is properly installed. The installation must meet the manufacturer's specified guidelines along with design changes at installation. Also, the supporting electrical utilities must meet all electrical codes. The information required for an IQ evaluation should be: equipment identification, required documentation, equipment utility requirements, major component specifications, component material, lubricants and equipment safety features.

5.1 Equipment Identification

Record the equipment identification numbers in Table I, along with the following information: equipment manufacturer, purchase order number, model number, serial number, company assigned equipment number, and the location of the equipment.

Writing Tip: The following information is found on the nameplate (placard) attached to the equipment and the equipment manufacturer's installation and operations manual.

Table I Equipment Identification

Required Information	As-found Conditions
Manufacturer	Any Mixer Co.
Purchase Order Number	004482
Model Number	Series 001 Model MC 501
Serial Number	55356 B
Equipment Number	2052
Location	Room 802 (This equipment is portable.)

Performed By:	Date:
Verified By:	Date:

℞ **Equipment Qualification Protocol**	Protocol No.: 4010
Title: (Any Mixer Co.) Model ME501 Emulsifying Mixer	Page: 5 of 21

5.2   Required Documentation

Record the equipment manufacturer's operation and maintenance manual and drawings in Table II. Record the standard operating procedures that cover the setup, operation and cleaning of the mixer in Table III.

Table II   Required Documentation

Number	Description	Date
None	*Installation Operation Instructions*	*None*
D-1346	*Standard Production Mixer Emulsifier*	*1/4/83*

Table III   Standard Operating Procedures

Number	Description	Release Date
GRA025	Granulation Equipment Setup	10/23/92
GRA026	Granulation Department Equipment Cleaning Procedure	03/12/96

5.3   Equipment Utility Requirements

Compare the manufacturer's specified volt (V) and amps (A) requirements to their as-found condition at the time of qualification testing and record the results in Table IV. Also, record the location of the power supply source. Record the instrument used to measure the volts and amps in Table V.

Performed By:	Date:
Verified By:	Date:

℞ **Equipment Qualification Protocol**	Protocol No.: 4010
Title: (Any Mixer Co.) Model ME501 Emulsifying Mixer	Page: 6 of 21

Volt Calculation:

    Volt specification = 460 V ±10%
    ±10% of 460 = ±46
    460 + 46 = 506
    460 - 46 = 414
The measured volts of 461/468/466 fall within ±10%

Amp Calculation:

    Circuit rating = 20 A
    Equipment current draw = 12.2 A
The circuit amp rating of 20 is greater than the maximum current draw of the equipment

Table IV   Utilities

Utility	Specified	Measured Results	Acceptable (Yes/No)
Volts	460 ±10%	A-B 461 A-C 468 B-C 466	Yes
Amps	Motor = 12.2	20 Circuit Rating	Yes

Power supply source, breaker box BB1, wire numbers: 31, 33, 35.

Table V   Instrument Used

Test Instrument	Identification Number	Calibration Due Date
Multimeter	ME-025	04/19/97

Performed By:	Date:
Verified By:	Date:

Ŗ **Equipment Qualification Protocol**	Protocol No.: 4010
Title: (Any Mixer Co.) Model ME501 Emulsifying Mixer	Page: 7 of 21

5.4 Major Component Specifications

The section is used to verify that the mixer components purchased were delivered and installed. Record the major components in Table VI.

Table VI   Major Components

Components	As-found Conditions
Mixer Motor	Manufacturer: Any Motor Co. Model Number: ME 501 Serial Number: 55356 C Volts: 460 Amperes: 12.2 Phases: 3 Cycles: 60 Hz hp: 5 rpm: 3480
Shaft	Part Number: 45267 Size: 1/2" diameter by 36" long Material: 316 Stainless Steel
Impeller	Part Number: 45268 Size: 1/2" bore by 6" diameter Material: 316 Stainless Steel
Performed By:	Date:
Verified By:	Date:

℞ Equipment Qualification Protocol	Protocol No.: 4010
Title: (Any Mixer Co.) Model ME501 Emulsifying Mixer	Page: 8 of 21

5.5 Component Material

Record the material of each component that contacts the product in Table VII.

Table VII Component Material

Component	Material
Shaft	316 Stainless Steel
Impeller	316 Stainless Steel
Rotor Shaft Bushing	Teflon

5.6 Lubricants

Record the lubricant used to operate the mixer in Table VIII and indicate if they make contact with the product. Is there is a preventive maintenance procedure on file? (Yes/No) *Yes*

Table VIII Lubricants

Where Used	Type	Manufacturer	Product Contact (Yes/No)
Motor Bearings	Lubriplate 630 AA	Any Oil Co.	No

5.7 Equipment Safety Features

The mixer is used in an explosive atmosphere. There are no safety features on this equipment. Nevertheless, there are some general safety precautions that should be followed when operating a mixer.

Performed By:	Date:
Verified By:	Date:

℞ **Equipment Qualification Protocol**	Protocol No.: 4010
Title: (Any Mixer Co.) Model ME501 Emulsifying Mixer	Page: 9 of 21

- Never touch a mixer, which has an electric motor, or any part of an electrical service line cord with wet hands or wet feet or if standing on a wet surface.

- Never attempt to move or adjust a mixer while it is running.

- Never touch any rotating part of a mixer with bare hands, gloved hands or with any hand-held object. Rotating parts include, but are not limited to, the mixer shaft, impeller(s), mechanical seals and motor fans.

- Do not touch a mixer motor until it cools. The motor temperature may be high enough to cause burns to the hands.

6.0   Operational Qualification (OQ)

An OQ evaluation should establish that the equipment can operate within specified tolerances and limits. The mechanical ranges of the mixer are being challenged along with the basic mixer operations. The mixer will be validated for its operating ability, not how well it mixes liquids or powders. The information required for the OQ evaluation should be: calibration of the instrument used to control the mixer, equipment control functions (switches and pushbuttons) and equipment operation (mixer rotation direction and mixer speed).

6.1   Calibration Requirements

Verify that all critical instruments on the equipment are logged into the calibration system, have calibration procedures in place and are currently in calibration at the time of qualification testing. Record all of the necessary information for the calibrated instruments used to control the mixer in Table IX.

Performed By:	Date:
Verified By:	Date:

R Equipment Qualification Protocol	Protocol No.: 4010
Title: (Any Mixer Co.) Model ME501 Emulsifying Mixer	Page: 10 of 21

Table IX   Calibrated and Non Calibrated Instruments

There were no calibrated or non calibrated instruments on this equipment.

Instrument	As-found Conditions
None	

6.2   Equipment Control Functions

Test Objective. The objective of this test is to verify that the switches on the mixer operate per manufacturer specifications. The mixer will be operated with the impeller submerged in water. The controls that need to be tested are: On Switch and Off Switch.

Test Procedure.

Materials and instruments required: mixing container, test fluid

- Fill the mixing container with water to its maximum working volume of 103 L and record the amount used in Table X. When operating the mixer the head must be submerged in the water to prevent damage to the mixer.

Test Fluid Volume Calculation:

Test fluid volume $= 75\%$ of 138 L $= 103.5$ L (rounded off to 103 L)

- Press the On Switch and verify that the mixer starts operating then record the results in Table XI.

Prepared By:	Date:
Verified By:	Date:

R Equipment Qualification Protocol	Protocol No.: 4010
Title: (Any Mixer Co.) Model ME501 Emulsifying Mixer	Page: 11 of 21

- Press the Off Switch and verify that the mixer stops operating then record the results in Table XI.

Table X   Test Materials

Item	Results
Mixing Container	138 L
Test Fluid	Water
Test Fluid Volume	103 L

Table XI   Control Function Test Results

Test Function	Expected Results	Acceptable (Yes/No)
Start Switch Operation	When the Start Switch is pressed, the mixer starts.	Yes
Stop Switch Operation	When the Stop Switch is pressed, the mixer stops.	Yes

6.3   Equipment Operation

6.3.1   Mixer Rotation Direction Test

Test Objective. The objective of this test is to verify that the mixer motor rotates in the proper direction. The mixer will be operated with the impeller being submerged in water.

Prepared By:	Date:
Verified By:	Date:

Ɍ **Equipment Qualification Protocol**	Protocol No.: 4010
Title: (Any Mixer Co.) Model ME501 Emulsifying Mixer	Page: 12 of 21

Test Procedure

Materials and instruments required: mixing container, test fluid

- Fill the mixing container with water to its maximum working volume of 103 L and record the amount used in Table XII. When operating the mixer the head must be submerged in the water to prevent damage to the mixer.

Test fluid volume calculation:

Test fluid volume = 75% of 138 L = 103.5 L (rounded off to 103 L)

- Press the Start key and observe the direction of rotation of the mixer motor as viewed from the top of the mixer and record the results in Table XIII.

Table XII   Test Materials

Item	Results
Mixing Container	138 L
Test Fluid	Water
Test Fluid Volume	103 L

Table XIII   Mixer Motor Rotation Direction Test Results

Item	Expected Results	Results	Acceptable (Yes/No)
Mixer Motor Rotation Direction	Rotation should be clockwise as viewed from the top of the mixer.	Clockwise rotation was observed.	Yes
Prepared By:			Date:
Verified By:			Date:

℞ **Equipment Qualification Protocol**	Protocol No.: 4010
Title: (Any Mixer Co.) Model ME501 Emulsifying Mixer	Page: 13 of 21

6.3.2   Mixer Speed Test

The speed test will not be performed during the OQ because the mixer cannot be operated without the impeller being submerged in water or other representative fluid or powder. This test is being performed in the PQ.

7.0   Performance Qualification (PQ)

Once it has been established that the equipment is properly installed and functioning within specified operating parameters, it must be shown that the mixer can be operated reliably under routine, minimum and maximum operating conditions.

7.1   Emulsifying Mixer Operation

Test Objective. The objective of this test is to document the performance of the mixer using water and a colored dye. Water will be used for maximum loading conditions. Also, the objective of this test is to verify that the mixer can move the fluid about the container (i.e., mixing). The speed of the mixer will be measured and recorded.

Test Procedure

Materials and instruments required: mixing container, test fluid, dye, tachometer

* Fill the mixing container with water to its maximum working volume of 103 L and record the amount used in Table XIV. When operating the mixer the head must be submerged in the water to prevent damage to the mixer.

   Test Fluid Volume Calculation:

   Test fluid volume = 75% of 138 L = 103.5 L (rounded off to 103 L)

Prepared By:	Date:
Verified By:	Date:

R **Equipment Qualification Protocol**	Protocol No.: 4010
Title: (Any Mixer Co.) Model ME501 Emulsifying Mixer	Page: 14 of 21

- Turn the mixer on and observe the motion of the fluid and record the results in Table XV. The results of this test are qualitative only and are based on observation.

- Add FDC blue #1 dye to the water and observe the mixing action of the mixer and record the results in Table XV. Verify that the added dye is distributed uniformly throughout the container. Record the dye used in Table XIV.

- Measure the speed of the mixer with a calibrated tachometer. Verify that the measured speed is within $\pm 10\%$ of the fixed speed of 3480 rpm. Record the results in Table XVI and the instrument used to measure the speed in Table XVII.

Mixer Speed Calculation:

Mixer speed specification = 3480 rpm $\pm 10\%$
$\pm 10\%$ of 3480 = ± 348
3480 + 348 = 3828
3480 - 348 = 3132
The measured rpm of 3521 falls within $\pm 10\%$

Table XIV   Test Materials

Item	Results
Mixing Container	138 L
Test Fluid	Water
Dye	FDC Blue #1
Test Fluid Volume	103 L

Prepared By:	Date:
Verified By:	Date:

℞ **Equipment Qualification Protocol**	Protocol No.: 4010	
Title: (Any Mixer Co.) Model ME501 Emulsifying Mixer		Page: 15 of 21

Table XV Mixer Performance Test Results

Test Function	Expected Results	Results	Acceptable (Yes/No)
Fluid Mixing Capabilities	The mixer should move the fluid about the container.	Fluid motion and vortex action was observed. There was increased motion with increased speed. *	Yes
Fluid Mixing Capabilities	The added dye should be distributed uniformly throughout the container.	The dye was distributed uniformly throughout the container. *	Yes

* The results of this test are qualitative only, and are based on observation.

Table XVI Mixer Speed Test Results

Item	Specification rpm	Measured Speed rpm	Acceptable (Yes/No)
Mixer Speed	3480 ±10%	3521	Yes

Table XVII Instrument Used

Test Instrument	Identification Number	Calibration Due Date
Tachometer	64020	06/21/97

Prepared By:		Date:
Verified By:		Date:

℞ **Equipment Qualification Protocol**	Protocol No.: 4010
Title: (Any Mixer Co.) Model ME501 Emulsifying Mixer	Page: 16 of 21

Attachment 1

Equipment Critical Instruments and
Test Equipment Calibration Certifications

℞ **Equipment Qualification Protocol**	Protocol No.: 4010
Title: (Any Mixer Co.) Model ME501 Emulsifying Mixer	Page: 17 of 21

Attachment 2

Calculation or Data Sheets

Ŗ Equipment Qualification Protocol	Protocol No.: 4010
Title: (Any Mixer Co.) Model ME501 Emulsifying Mixer	Page: 18 of 21

Attachment 3

Test Results

℞ **Equipment Qualification Protocol**	Protocol No.: 4010
Title: (Any Mixer Co.) Model ME501 Emulsifying Mixer	Page: 19 of 21

Attachment 4

Preventive Maintenance Schedule

R̶ **Equipment Qualification Protocol**	Protocol No.: 4010
Title: (Any Mixer Co.) Model ME501 Emulsifying Mixer	Page: 20 of 21

Attachment 5

Deficiencies

R̶ **Equipment Qualification Protocol**	Protocol No.: 4010
Title: (Any Mixer Co.) Model ME501 Emulsifying Mixer	Page: 21 of 21

Attachment 6

Placebo Batch Records

See Chapter 6 under "Deficiency" for information on how to develop and use a deficiency form.

℞	**Deficiency Form**	
Prepared by:	Date: 10/17/98	DF No.: 001

Title: (Any Mixer Co.) Model ME501 Emulsifying Mixer

The deficiency is: Non-Critical ❏ Critical ☒

Affected Dept(s).: R&D and Operations

Describe the Deficiency: (Reference: Page 25 of Protocol 4025)
The cooling supply's water pressure was measured at 62 psig which is greater than the manufacturer's specification of ≤30 psig for the Bowl Jacket and ≤10 psig for the Washdown Valves. There is not a pressure regulator on the supply line.

Describe the impact if this deficiency is not corrected:
Blockage in the drain line could cause the water pressure in the Bowl Jacket to exceed the Jacket rating of ≤ 30 psig and the ≤ 10 psig for the Washdown Valves.

Correction Action:
Work Request No. 53115 was prepared by Maintenance for corrective action. A water pressure regulator will be installed on the water supply line.

Approved By:	
Validation Manager:	Date:
Maintenance:	Date:

See Chapter 6 under "Addendum" for information on how to develop and use an addendum.

R͗	**Addendum**		
Protocol Number: 4067 Title: (Any Labeler Co.) Plastic Bottle Labeler Model 112-PB			Addendum No.: A001
Manufacturer: Any Labeler Co.			Page: 1 of 2
Model Number: 112-PB		Serial Number: 2700D79M	
Equipment Number: 245		Location: Packaging Line 9	
Prepared By:			
Validation:			Date:
Approved By:			
Validation Manager:			Date:
Research & Development:			Date:
Operations:			Date:
Maintenance:			Date:
Regulatory Compliance:			Date:

R̸	Addendum	
Protocol Number: 4067		Addendum No.: A001
Title: (Any Labeler Co.) Plastic Bottle Labeler Model 112-PB		Page: 2 of 2

Operational Qualification

Imprinter Operation

Objective

The objective of this addendum is to add the qualification testing of the imprinter to the original validation. The imprinter was not validated because it was not ever used. It has been determined that there is a need for this function.

Method

- Visually observe 100 connective 1 3/4" x 3 3/8" size labels as they pass through imprinter and verify that 100% of the labels have a serial number and date printed on them. Record the results in the following Table I.

- Visually observe 100 connective 2 1/2" x 6" size labels as they pass through imprinter and verify that 100% of the labels have a serial number and date printed on them. Record the results in the following Table I.

Table I   Imprinter Test Results

Test	Number of Labels	Label Size	Number of Labels Imprinted	Acceptable (Yes/No)
1	100	1 3/4" x 3 3/8"	100	Yes
2	100	2 1/2" x 6"	100	Yes

Performed By:		Date:
Verified By:		Date:

Appendix E

Computer Qualification Protocol Example

I have included an actual qualification protocol template that is filled in to show you an example of how to develop a computer qualification protocol. Each of the protocol elements is covered in the template. This example illustrates a situation in which a computer is used to control case labeling print and apply systems on nine packaging lines. Only the computer qualification is shown in this example because each of the packaging line print and apply units is covered in equipment qualification protocols.

R̠	**Computer Qualification Protocol**	
Title: (Any Computer Co.) Model 575 Computer		Protocol No.: 5048
Manufacturer: Any Computer Co.		Page: 1 of 62
Model Number: 575	Serial Number: 74193	
Computer Number: 745	Location: Label Room	

Prepared By:		
Validation:		Date:
Approved By:		
Validation Manager:		Date:
Research & Development:		Date:
Operations:		Date:
Maintenance:		Date:
Regulatory Compliance:		Date:

R̥ Computer Qualification Protocol	Protocol No.: 5048
Title: (Any Computer Co.) Model 575 Computer	Page: 2 of 62

1.0 Table of Contents

R̥ **Computer Qualification Protocol**	Protocol No.: 5048
Title: (Any Computer Co.) Model 575 Computer	Page: 3 of 62

2.0   Objective

The objective of this Computer qualification is to establish documented evidence that the computer and print and apply system is acceptably installed per manufacturer recommendations, process requirements, and/or engineering standards. Acceptable installation includes suitable utility connections, components, and critical instruments in current calibration. Acceptable operation includes, as applicable, proper control and sequencing functions, recording and reporting functions, and safety and alarm features that meet process requirements and equipment specifications. Acceptable performance includes consistent operation within specified process parameters under simulated or actual production conditions.

3.0   Scope

The scope of this computer qualification protocol includes the computer and print and apply system and its associated components. Installation qualification is limited to the system components and does not include installation of support utilities, other than the connections at the system boundary. Operational testing is limited to demonstrating computer functionality. Product specific testing is outside the scope of this qualification document, other than where a product is used to demonstrate computer functionality.

4.0   Computer and Print and Apply System Description

The print and apply system is provided by (any print and apply co.). The system consists of a PC with software and a back-up PC with software. The PCs are interfaced with each of 9 packaging lines, containing (any software companies) software and a label printer and a deskjet printer. The equipment located at the end of each packaging line consists of a conveyor belt, print and apply equipment, a scanner to scan the label barcode, a decoder to compare the barcode scanned to the barcode entered at the PC, and an indicator light.

R̥ **Computer Qualification Protocol**	Protocol No.: 5048
Title: (Any Computer Co.) Model 575 Computer	Page: 4 of 62

4.0   Computer and Print and Apply System Description (Continued.)

The system is used to print case labels on the packaging line, apply the printed label to the case as it travels down the conveyor belt, and then scan the barcode on the label, ensuring the label contains the correct barcode for the product being run. The system also provides online monitoring of each of the packaging lines. Label Room operators can view the Data Monitoring screen on the PC and tell which lines are operating, how close a print job is to completion, whether a line is stopped, whether a print job has been terminated before completion, and if a print job has been restarted.

In the Label Room, a data file containing the product numbers, the product names, and case package sizes, along with the key fields and item numbers is imported into the software. This imported file is created from a file generated by company product database. Using MS-Access, the format of the file is modified so that it can be imported into the Case Labeling software. A Label Room operator selects the item number for the product being run from the main screen and either selects or types in the necessary information for the Batch number, Expiration Date, Case Size, Quantity, and Packaging Line. A test label is printed on the label printer in the Label Room and verified by the operator. If any of the information is incorrect on the label, it can be re-entered and a new test label printed. Once the label is verified, the print job is sent to the packaging line specified in the main screen. The Label Room operators will monitor the status of the Case Labeling System from the Status Update screen. The Label Issuance operators may clear a print job and print a Production Report.

At the packaging line, the packaging line operators place a case containing product on the conveyor belt. The case travels down the conveyor belt under the Belt Hold down unit. A photocell alerts the print and apply station that a case is on the conveyor belt and to print a label. The label is printed and then held in place on the perforated applicator roller by suction created by compressed air flowing through the roller. As the case passes by the label applicator, the label is applied to the case. The case travels further down the conveyor belt where the barcode is scanned. If the barcode is incorrect or the scanner is unable to get a good scan of the label, the conveyor belt shuts down and the red indicator light flashes, notifying the packaging line operator of a problem. If the barcode is scanned and determined to be correct by the decoder, the case is allowed to continue down the line.

℞ **Computer Qualification Protocol**	Protocol No.: 5048
Title: (Any Computer Co.) Model 575 Computer	Page: 5 of 62

5.0   Installation Qualification (IQ)

An IQ evaluation will establish confidence that the computer and print and apply system is properly installed. The installation must meet the manufacturer's specified guidelines along with design changes at installation. Also, the supporting electrical utilities must meet all electrical codes. The information required for an IQ evaluation should be: computer identification, required documentation, computer utility requirements, major component specifications, component material, lubricants and computer safety features.

5.1   Computer Identification

Record the Computer identification numbers in Table I, along with the following information: Computer manufacturer, purchase order number, model number, serial number, company assigned equipment number, and the location of the Computer.

Writing Tip: The following information is found on the nameplate (placard) attached to the Computer and the Computer manufacturer's installation and operations manual.

Table I   Computer System Identification

Required Information	As-found Conditions
Manufacturer	Any Computer Co.
Purchase Order Number	075139
Model Number	575
Serial Number	74193
Computer Number	575
Location	Label Room

Performed By:	Date:
Verified By:	Date:

Ŗ **Computer Qualification Protocol**	Protocol No.: 5048
Title: (Any Computer Co.) Model 575 Computer	Page: 6 of 62

5.2   Required Documentation

Record the computer and print and apply equipment manufacturer's operation and maintenance manual and drawings in Table II. Record the standard operating procedures that cover the setup, operation and cleaning of the computer in Table III.

Table II   Required Documentation

Number	Description	Date
29700	Installation and Operation Instructions	07/15/98
297001	Print and Apply System Software Manual	09/08/88

Table III   Standard Operating Procedures

Number	Description	Release Date
PKG025	Computer and Print and Apply System Setup	10/23/97
PKG026	Print and Apply Equipment Cleaning Procedure	03/12/97

5.3   Computer Utility Requirements

Compare the manufacturer's specified volt (V) and amps (A) requirements to their as-found condition at the time of qualification testing and record the results in Table IV. Also, record the location of the power supply source. Record the instrument used to measure the volts and amps in Table V.

Performed By:	Date:
Verified By:	Date:

℞ **Computer Qualification Protocol**	Protocol No.: 5048
Title: (Any Computer Co.) Model 575 Computer	Page: 7 of 62

Volt Calculation:

    Volt specification = 115 V ±10%
±10% of 115 = ±11.5
115 + 11.5 = 126.5
115 − 11.5 = 103.5
The measured volts of 114 fall within ±10%

Amp Calculation:

    Circuit rating = 20 A
Computer current draw = 6 A
The circuit amp rating of 20 is greater than the maximum current draw of the Computer

Table IV   Utilities

Utility	Specified	Measured Results	Acceptable (Yes/No)
Volts	115 ±10%	114	Yes
Amps	6	20 Circuit Rating	Yes

Power supply source, breaker box BB1, wire number: 3.

Table V   Instrument Used

Test Instrument	Identification Number	Calibration Due Date
Multimeter	ME-025	04/19/97

Performed By:	Date:
Verified By:	Date:

℞ **Computer Qualification Protocol**	Protocol No.: 5048
Title: (Any Computer Co.) Model 575 Computer	Page: 8 of 62

5.4   Major Component Specifications

The section is used to verify that the computer system components purchased were delivered and installed. Record the major components in Table VI.

Table VI   Major Components

Components	As-found Conditions
Personal Computer Hardware Processor Main Memory Disk Space Monitor Ports Mouse Printer	Personal Computer Hardware Pentium (r) 64 MB RAM 1 GB VGA 3 COM Ports Mouse Laserjet or Postscript
Personal Computer (Back-up) Hardware Processor Main Memory Disk Space Monitor Ports Mouse Printer	Personal Computer Hardware Pentium (r) 64 MB RAM 1 GB VGA 3 COM Ports Mouse Laserjet or Postscript
Performed By:	Date:
Verified By:	Date:

R Computer Qualification Protocol		Protocol No.: 5048
Title: (Any Computer Co.) Model 575 Computer		Page: 9 of 62

Table VI   Major Components (Continued.)

Components	As-found Conditions
Personal Computer Software MS Windows 95 Performance Series Product Labeling Manager	Personal Computer Software Version 4.00 or higher Version 1.7 Version 1.0.0
Personal Computer (Back-up) Software MS Windows 95 Performance Series Product Labeling Manager	Personal Computer Software Version 4.00 or higher Version 1.7 Version 1.0.0
Performance Series Software Diskettes, version 1.7 Manual	2 diskettes in Facility Services Manual in Packaging Library
Product labeling manager Version 1.3	1 diskette stored in the Packaging Engineer's Office
DeskJet Page Printer	HP Deskjet 550C
Diagraph Label Printing System Performance Series	Fargo Prodigy Plus 8
Diagraph Label Printing System Performance Series (Backup)	Fargo Prodigy Plus 8
Code-Activated Switch Box	Wti CAS-161A

Performed By:		Date:
Verified By:		Date:

℞ **Computer Qualification Protocol**	Protocol No.: 5048
Title: (Any Computer Co.) Model 575 Computer	Page: 10 of 62

5.5   Component/Subsystem Configuration

Objective

The objective of this procedure is to document the current configuration of the computerized system including: configurable hardware parameters, directory and file structure listings for the PC hard drive, and critical start-up software. This will provide a configuration baseline of the system at the time of qualification testing.

Procedure

Document pertinent (non-standard) configurable parameters and executable files for the PC. Record the location, byte size and date of the system start-up files and software currently stored on the hard drive of the PC in Table VII. Include a printout of the hard drive directory listings and system startup files (autoexec.bat) in Attachment 1.

Acceptance Criteria

All pertinent, non-standard hardware and software parameters are documented for baseline information only.

Performed By:	Date:
Verified By:	Date:

℞ **Computer Qualification Protocol**	Protocol No.: 5048
Title: (Any Computer Co.) Model 575 Computer	Page: 11 of 62

Acceptance Criteria (Continued.)

Table VII Non-Standard Configuration Parameters

Software			
Program or File Name	**Location/Path**	**Byte Size**	**Date**
Autoexec.bat	C:\	1 KB	04/27/98
Digicard Terminals	C:\	125 KB	05/18/98
Plblman	C:\	1563 KB	05/30/98
Back-up Computer			
Autoexec.bat	C:\	1 KB	04/27/98
Digicard Terminals	C:\	1125 KB	05/18/98
Plblman	C:\	1563 KB	05/30/98

Performed By:	Date:
Verified By:	Date:

R **Computer Qualification Protocol**	Protocol No.: 5048
Title: (Any Computer Co.) Model 575 Computer	Page: 12 of 62

5.6   Component Material

Record the material of each component that contacts the product in Table VIII.

Table VIII   Component Material

Component	Material
None.	

5.7   Lubricants

Record the lubricant used to operate the computer in Table IX and indicate if they make contact with the product. Is there is a preventive maintenance procedure on file? (Yes/No) Yes.

Table IX   Lubricants

Where Used	Type	Manufacturer	Product Contact (Yes/No)
None.			

5.8   Computer Safety Features

There are no safety features on the computer system.

Performed By:	Date:
Verified By:	Date:

Ŗ **Computer Qualification Protocol**	Protocol No.: 5048
Title: (Any Computer Co.) Model 575 Computer	Page: 13 of 62

6.0   Operational Qualification (OQ)

An OQ evaluation should establish that the computer system can operate within specified tolerances and limits. The mechanical ranges of the computer are being challenged along with the basic computer operations. The information required for the OQ evaluation should be: calibration of the instrument used to control the computer, computer control functions (switches and pushbuttons) and computer operation.

6.1   Calibration Requirements

Verify that all critical instruments on the computer are logged into the calibration system, have calibration procedures in place and are currently in calibration at the time of qualification testing. Record all of the necessary information for the calibrated instruments used to control the computer in Table X.

Table X   Calibrated and Non Calibrated Instruments

There were no calibrated or non calibrated instruments on this Computer.

Instrument	As-found Conditions
None.	

Performed By:		Date:
Verified By:		Date:

R	Computer Qualification Protocol	Protocol No.: 5048

Title: (Any Computer Co.) Model 575 Computer	Page: 14 of 62

6.2 Control Functions

Objective. To verify that the pull-down menus and buttons perform as expected. In the Results column, specify "AE" for "as expected" or if not enter information.

Item No.	Expected Results	Results	Acceptable (Yes/No)
MAIN MENU - View Only User			
1	After selecting Product Labeling Manager from the Start push-up menu, the main screen displays (8) Pull Down Menus: File, View, Tools (grayed out), Data (grayed out), Security, User (grayed out), Configure (grayed out), and Help. Also displayed are the (10) Buttons: Rx, Open Book, Open Calendar, Key, Hand (grayed out), Pages Plus Arrow-Left (grayed out), Pages Plus Arrow-Right (grayed out), Rx (grayed out), X (grayed out), and Magnifying Glass (grayed out). Also displayed is the Status Bar.	AE	Yes
2	After selecting the File Pull-Down Menu (1) option is displayed: Exit (grayed out).	AE	Yes
3	After selecting Exit, nothing happens.	AE	Yes
4	After selecting the View Pull-Down Menu (5) options are displayed: Toolbar (with a check mark in front of it), Status Bar (with a check mark in front of it), View Product Data, Job Status and Job History.	AE	Yes

Performed By:	Date:
Verified By:	Date:

R̶x̶	**Computer Qualification Protocol**	Protocol No.: 5048

Title: (Any Computer Co.) Model 575 Computer	Page: 15 of 62

6.2 Control Functions (Continued.)

Item No.	Expected Results	Results	Acceptable (Yes/No)
	**MAIN MENU - View Only User** (Continued.)		
5	After selecting Toolbar, the Toolbar disappears. After selecting Toolbar again, the Toolbar reappears.	AE	Yes
6	After selecting Status Bar, the Status Bar disappears. After selecting the Status Bar again the Status Bar reappears.	AE	Yes
7	After selecting View Product Data, the View Product Data Window is displayed and (1) button: Close.	AE	Yes
8	After Close is selected the Product Labeling Manager screen is displayed.	AE	Yes
9	After selecting Job Status, the Job Status window is displayed and (4) Buttons are displayed: Pause, Refresh, Start and Close.	AE	Yes
10	After selecting Pause, the window remains the same without updates allowing the user to scroll left and right without refreshing the screen.	AE	Yes
11	After selecting Refresh, the window will be updated.	AE	Yes
12	After selecting Start, the window will return to updating data at set intervals.	AE	Yes

Performed By:	Date:
Verified By:	Date:

℞ **Computer Qualification Protocol**		Protocol No.: 5048	
Title: (Any Computer Co.) Model 575 Computer			Page: 16 of 62

6.2 Control Functions (Continued.)

Item No.	Expected Results	Results	Acceptable (Yes/No)
MAIN MENU - View Only User (Continued.)			
13	After selecting Close, the Product Labeling Manager Main screen is displayed.	AE	Yes
14	After selecting View Drop-Down Menu, the Job History window is displayed and (1) Button: Close.	AE	Yes
15	After selecting Close, the Product Labeling Manager screen is displayed.	AE	Yes
16	After selecting the (grayed out) Tools Drop-Down Menu, nothing happens.	AE	Yes
17	After selecting the Security Drop-Down Menu, (2) options are displayed: Logon/Logoff, Administer (grayed out).	AE	Yes
18	After selecting Logon/Logoff, the Logon/Logoff window is displayed and (2) Buttons: OK, Cancel.	AE	Yes
19	After selecting the arrow in the User Name box, (3) options are displayed: Administrator, Supervisor, and User.	AE	Yes
20	After selecting the OK Button, the selection is accepted.	AE	Yes
21	After selecting Cancel, the Product Labeling Manager screen is displayed.	AE	Yes
Performed By:		Date:	
Verified By:		Date:	

℞ **Computer Qualification Protocol**		Protocol No.: 5048	
Title: (Any Computer Co.) Model 575 Computer			Page: 17 of 62

6.2 Control Functions (Continued.)

Item No.	Expected Results	Results	Acceptable (Yes/No)
MAIN MENU - View Only User (Continued.)			
22	After selecting the (grayed out) User Pull-Down menu, nothing happens.	AE	Yes
23	After selecting the (grayed out) Configure Pull-Down menu, nothing happens.	AE	Yes
24	After selecting the Help Pull-Down Menu, (2) options are displayed: Contents and About.	AE	Yes
25	After selecting Contents, a secondary Drop-Down Menu is displayed with (2) options: Extract Help Files and View On-Line Help.	AE	Yes
26	After selecting Extract Help Files, the On-Line Help Window is displayed and (1) Button: OK.	AE	Yes
27	After selecting OK, the Product Labeling Manager screen is displayed.	AE	Yes
28	After selecting View, then View On-Line Help, the Frameset 1- Microsoft Internet Explorer Window with the Table of Contents for the Product Labeling Manager Program is displayed.	AE	Yes
29	After selecting the X Button in the upper right corner, the Product Labeling Manager screen is displayed.	AE	Yes

Performed By:		Date:
Verified By:		Date:

R Computer Qualification Protocol			Protocol No.: 5048	
Title: (Any Computer Co.) Model 575 Computer				Page: 18 of 62

6.2 **Control Functions** (Continued.)

Item No.	Expected Results	Results	Acceptable (Yes/No)
MAIN MENU - View Only User (Continued.)			
30	After selecting the Rx Button (Left side of screen), the Product Data Window is displayed and (1) Button: Close.	AE	Yes
31	After selecting the Close Button, the Product Labeling Manager screen is displayed.	AE	Yes
32	After selecting the Open Book Button, the Current Job Status Window is displayed.	AE	Yes
33	After selecting Pause, the window remains the same without updates allowing the user to scroll left and right without refreshing the screen.	AE	Yes
34	After selecting Refresh, the window will be updated.	AE	Yes
35	After selecting Start, the window will return to updating data at set intervals.	AE	Yes
36	After selecting Close, the Product Labeling Manager Main screen is displayed.	AE	Yes
37	After selecting Open Calendar Button, the Job History Window is displayed and (1) Button: Close.	AE	Yes
38	After selecting the Close Button, the Product Labeling Manager screen is displayed.	AE	Yes

Performed By:	Date:
Verified By:	Date:

R̟ **Computer Qualification Protocol**	Protocol No.: 5048

Title: (Any Computer Co.) Model 575 Computer	Page: 19 of 62

6.2   Control Functions (Continued.)

Item No.	Expected Results	Results	Acceptable (Yes/No)
MAIN MENU - View Only User (Continued.)			
39	After selecting the Key Button, the Logon/Logoff Window is displayed.	AE	Yes
40	After selecting the arrow in the User Name box, (3) options are displayed: Administrator, Supervisor, and User.	AE	Yes
41	After selecting the OK Button, the selection is accepted.	AE	Yes
42	After selecting Cancel, the Product Labeling Manager screen is displayed.	AE	Yes
43	After selecting the (grayed out) Hand Button, nothing happens.	AE	Yes
44	After selecting the (grayed out) Pages Plus Arrow-Left Button, nothing happens.	AE	Yes
45	After selecting the (grayed out) Pages Plus Arrow-Right Button, nothing happens.	AE	Yes
46	After selecting the (grayed out) Rx Button, nothing happens.	AE	Yes
47	After selecting the (grayed out) X (Clear Buffer) Button, nothing happens.	AE	Yes
48	After selecting the (grayed out) Magnifying Glass, nothing happens.	AE	Yes

Performed By:	Date:
Verified By:	Date:

R **Computer Qualification Protocol**		Protocol No.: 5048	
Title: (Any Computer Co.) Model 575 Computer			Page: 20 of 62

6.2   Control Functions (Continued.)

Item No.	Expected Results	Results	Acceptable (Yes/No)
MAIN MENU - User			
1	After selecting Product Labeling Manager from the Start push-up menu, the main screen displays (8) Pull Down Menus: File, View, Tools (grayed out), Data (grayed out), Security, User (grayed out), Configure (grayed out), and Help. Also displayed are the (10) Buttons: Rx, Open Book, Open Calendar, Key, Hand (grayed out), Pages Plus Arrow-Left (grayed out), Pages Plus Arrow-Right (grayed out), Rx (grayed out), X (grayed out), and Magnifying Glass (grayed out). Also displayed is the Status Bar.	AE	Yes
2	After selecting the File Pull-Down Menu (1) option is displayed: Exit (grayed out).	AE	Yes
3	After selecting Exit, nothing happens.	AE	Yes
4	After selecting the View Pull-Down Menu (5) options are displayed: Toolbar (with a check mark in front of it), Status Bar (with a check mark in front of it), View Product Data, Job Status and Job History.	AE	Yes

Performed By:	Date:
Verified By:	Date:

R̶ Computer Qualification Protocol		Protocol No.: 5048	
Title: (Any Computer Co.) Model 575 Computer			Page: 21 of 62

6.2 Control Functions (Continued.)

Item No.	Expected Results	Results	Acceptable (Yes/No)
MAIN MENU - User (Continued.)			
5	After selecting Toolbar, the Toolbar disappears. After selecting Toolbar again, the Toolbar reappears.	AE	Yes
6	After selecting Status Bar, the Status Bar disappears. After selecting the Status Bar again the Status Bar reappears.	AE	Yes
7	After selecting View Product Data, the View Product Data Window is displayed and (1) button: Close.	AE	Yes
8	After Close is selected the Product Labeling Manager screen is displayed.	AE	Yes
9	After selecting Job Status, the Job Status window is displayed and (4) Buttons are displayed: Pause, Refresh, Start and Close.	AE	Yes
10	After selecting Pause, the window remains the same without updates allowing the user to scroll left and right without refreshing the screen.	AE	Yes
11	After selecting Refresh, the window will be updated.	AE	Yes
12	After selecting Start, the window will return to updating data at set intervals.	AE	Yes
Performed By:		Date:	
Verified By:		Date:	

R **Computer Qualification Protocol**		Protocol No.: 5048	
Title: (Any Computer Co.) Model 575 Computer			Page: 22 of 62

6.2   Control Functions (Continued.)

Item No.	Expected Results	Results	Acceptable (Yes/No)
MAIN MENU - User (Continued.)			
13	After selecting Close, the Product Labeling Manager Main screen is displayed.	AE	Yes
14	After selecting View Drop-Down Menu, the Job History window is displayed and (1) Button: Close.	AE	Yes
15	After selecting Close, the Product Labeling Manager screen is displayed.	AE	Yes
16	After selecting the (grayed out) Tools Drop-Down Menu, nothing happens.	AE	Yes
17	After selecting the Security Drop-Down Menu, (2) options are displayed: Logon/Logoff, Administer (grayed out).	AE	Yes
18	After selecting Logon/Logoff, the Logon/Logoff window is displayed and (2) Buttons: OK, Cancel.	AE	Yes
19	After selecting the arrow in the User Name box, (3) options are displayed: Administrator, Supervisor, and User.	AE	Yes
20	After selecting the OK Button, the selection is accepted.	AE	Yes
21	After selecting Cancel, the Product Labeling Manager screen is displayed.	AE	Yes

Performed By:		Date:
Verified By:		Date:

℞	**Computer Qualification Protocol**	Protocol No.: 5048

Title: (Any Computer Co.) Model 575 Computer	Page: 23 of 62

6.2 Control Functions (Continued.)

Item No.	Expected Results	Results	Acceptable (Yes/No)
\multicolumn{4}{l}{MAIN MENU - User (Continued.)}			
22	After selecting the (grayed out) User Pull-Down menu, nothing happens.	AE	Yes
23	After selecting the (grayed out) Configure Pull-Down menu, nothing happens.	AE	Yes
24	After selecting the Help Pull-Down Menu, (2) options are displayed: Contents and About.	AE	Yes
25	After selecting Contents, a secondary Drop-Down Menu is displayed with (2) options: Extract Help Files and View On-Line Help.	AE	Yes
26	After selecting Extract Help Files, the On-Line Help Window is displayed and (1) Button: OK.	AE	Yes
27	After selecting OK, the Product Labeling Manager screen is displayed.	AE	Yes
28	After selecting View, then View On-Line Help, the Frameset 1- Microsoft Internet Explorer Window with the Table of Contents for the Product Labeling Manager Program is displayed.	AE	Yes
29	After selecting the X Button in the upper right corner, the Product Labeling Manager screen is displayed.	AE	Yes

Performed By:	Date:
Verified By:	Date:

R	**Computer Qualification Protocol**	Protocol No.: 5048
Title: (Any Computer Co.) Model 575 Computer		Page: 24 of 62

6.2 Control Functions (Continued.)

Item No.	Expected Results	Results	Acceptable (Yes/No)
MAIN MENU - User (Continued.)			
30	After selecting the Rx Button (Left side of screen), the Product Data Window is displayed and (1) Button: Close.	AE	Yes
31	After selecting the Close Button, the Product Labeling Manager screen is displayed.	AE	Yes
32	After selecting the Open Book Button, the Current Job Status Window is displayed.	AE	Yes
33	After selecting Pause, the window remains the same without updates allowing the user to scroll left and right without refreshing the screen.	AE	Yes
34	After selecting Refresh, the window will be updated.	AE	Yes
35	After selecting Start, the window will return to updating data at set intervals.	AE	Yes
36	After selecting Close, the Product Labeling Manager Main screen is displayed.	AE	Yes
37	After selecting Open Calendar Button, the Job History Window is displayed and (1) Button: Close.	AE	Yes
38	After selecting the Close Button, the Product Labeling Manager screen is displayed.	AE	Yes
Performed By:		Date:	
Verified By:		Date:	

R	**Computer Qualification Protocol**	Protocol No.: 5048

Title: (Any Computer Co.) Model 575 Computer	Page: 25 of 62

6.2   Control Functions (Continued.)

Item No.	Expected Results	Results	Acceptable (Yes/No)
	MAIN MENU - User (Continued.)		
39	After selecting the Key Button, the Logon/Logoff Window is displayed.	AE	Yes
40	After selecting the arrow in the User Name box, (3) options are displayed: Administrator, Supervisor, and User.	AE	Yes
41	After selecting the OK Button, the selection is accepted.	AE	Yes
42	After selecting Cancel, the Product Labeling Manager screen is displayed.	AE	Yes
43	After selecting the (grayed out) Hand Button, nothing happens.	AE	Yes
44	After selecting the (grayed out) Pages Plus Arrow-Left Button, nothing happens.	AE	Yes
45	After selecting the (grayed out) Pages Plus Arrow-Right Button, nothing happens.	AE	Yes
46	After selecting the (grayed out) Rx Button, nothing happens.	AE	Yes
47	After selecting the (grayed out) X (Clear Buffer) Button, nothing happens.	AE	Yes
48	After selecting the (grayed out) Magnifying Glass, nothing happens.	AE	Yes

Performed By:	Date:
Verified By:	Date:

℞	**Computer Qualification Protocol**	Protocol No.: 5048
Title: (Any Computer Co.) Model 575 Computer		Page: 26 of 62

6.2 Control Functions (Continued.)

Item No.	Expected Results	Results	Acceptable (Yes/No)
MAIN MENU - Supervisor			
1	After selecting Product Labeling Manager from the Start push-up menu, the main screen displays (8) Pull Down Menus: File, View, Tools (grayed out), Data (grayed out), Security, User (grayed out), Configure (grayed out), and Help. Also displayed are the (10) Buttons: Rx, Open Book, Open Calendar, Key, Hand (grayed out), Pages Plus Arrow-Left (grayed out), Pages Plus Arrow-Right (grayed out), Rx (grayed out), X (grayed out), and Magnifying Glass (grayed out). Also displayed is the Status Bar.	AE	Yes
2	After selecting the File Pull-Down Menu (1) option is displayed: Exit (grayed out).	AE	Yes
3	After selecting Exit, nothing happens.	AE	Yes
4	After selecting the View Pull-Down Menu (5) options are displayed: Toolbar (with a check mark in front of it), Status Bar (with a checkmark in front of it), View Product Data, Job Status and Job History.	AE	Yes

Performed By:		Date:
Verified By:		Date:

R̞ Computer Qualification Protocol		Protocol No.: 5048
Title: (Any Computer Co.) Model 575 Computer		Page: 27 of 62

6.2   Control Functions (Continued.)

Item No.	Expected Results	Results	Acceptable (Yes/No)
MAIN MENU - Supervisor (Continued.)			
5	After selecting Toolbar, the Toolbar disappears. After selecting Toolbar again, the Toolbar reappears.	AE	Yes
6	After selecting Status Bar, the Status Bar disappears. After selecting the Status Bar again the Status Bar reappears.	AE	Yes
7	After selecting View Product Data, the View Product Data Window is displayed and (1) button: Close.	AE	Yes
8	After Close is selected the Product Labeling Manager screen is displayed.	AE	Yes
9	After selecting Job Status, the Job Status window is displayed and (4) Buttons are displayed: Pause, Refresh, Start and Close.	AE	Yes
10	After selecting Pause, the window remains the same without updates allowing the user to scroll left and right without refreshing the screen.	AE	Yes
11	After selecting Refresh, the window will be updated.	AE	Yes
12	After selecting Start, the window will return to updating data at set intervals.	AE	Yes
Performed By:		Date:	
Verified By:		Date:	

R Computer Qualification Protocol	Protocol No.: 5048

Title: (Any Computer Co.) Model 575 Computer	Page: 28 of 62

6.2 Control Functions (Continued.)

Item No.	Expected Results	Results	Acceptable (Yes/No)
MAIN MENU - Supervisor (Continued.)			
13	After selecting Close, the Product Labeling Manager Main screen is displayed.	AE	Yes
14	After selecting View Drop-Down Menu, the Job History window is displayed and (1) Button: Close.	AE	Yes
15	After selecting Close, the Product Labeling Manager screen is displayed.	AE	Yes
16	After selecting the (grayed out) Tools Drop-Down Menu, nothing happens.	AE	Yes
17	After selecting the Security Drop-Down Menu, (2) options are displayed: Logon/Logoff, Administer (grayed out).	AE	Yes
18	After selecting Logon/Logoff, the Logon/Logoff window is displayed and (2) Buttons: OK, Cancel.	AE	Yes
19	After selecting the arrow in the User Name box, (3) options are displayed: Administrator, Supervisor, and User.	AE	Yes
20	After selecting the OK Button, the selection is accepted.	AE	Yes
21	After selecting Cancel, the Product Labeling Manager screen is displayed.	AE	Yes

Performed By:	Date:
Verified By:	Date:

R̥ **Computer Qualification Protocol**		Protocol No.: 5048
Title: (Any Computer Co.) Model 575 Computer		Page: 29 of 62

6.2   Control Functions (Continued.)

Item No.	Expected Results	Results	Acceptable (Yes/No)
MAIN MENU - Supervisor (Continued.)			
22	After selecting the (grayed out) User Pull-Down menu, nothing happens.	AE	Yes
23	After selecting the (grayed out) Configure Pull-Down menu, nothing happens.	AE	Yes
24	After selecting the Help Pull-Down Menu, (2) options are displayed: Contents and About.	AE	Yes
25	After selecting Contents, a secondary Drop-Down Menu is displayed with (2) options: Extract Help Files and View On-Line Help.	AE	Yes
26	After selecting Extract Help Files, the On-Line Help Window is displayed and (1) Button: OK.	AE	Yes
27	After selecting OK, the Product Labeling Manager screen is displayed.	AE	Yes
28	After selecting View, then View On-Line Help, the Frameset 1- Microsoft Internet Explorer Window with the Table of Contents for the Product Labeling Manager Program is displayed.	AE	Yes
29	After selecting the X Button in the upper right corner, the Product Labeling Manager screen is displayed.	AE	Yes

Performed By:		Date:
Verified By:		Date:

R **Computer Qualification Protocol**		Protocol No.: 5048	
Title: (Any Computer Co.) Model 575 Computer			Page: 30 of 62

6.2 Control Functions (Continued.)

Item No.	Expected Results	Results	Acceptable (Yes/No)
MAIN MENU - Supervisor (Continued.)			
30	After selecting the Rx Button (Left side of screen), the Product Data Window is displayed and (1) Button: Close.	AE	Yes
31	After selecting the Close Button, the Product Labeling Manager screen is displayed.	AE	Yes
32	After selecting the Open Book Button, the Current Job Status Window is displayed.	AE	Yes
33	After selecting Pause, the window remains the same without updates allowing the user to scroll left and right without refreshing the screen.	AE	Yes
34	After selecting Refresh, the window will be updated.	AE	Yes
35	After selecting Start, the window will return to updating data at set intervals.	AE	Yes
36	After selecting Close, the Product Labeling Manager Main screen is displayed.	AE	Yes
37	After selecting Open Calendar Button, the Job History Window is displayed and (1) Button: Close.	AE	Yes
38	After selecting the Close Button, the Product Labeling Manager screen is displayed.	AE	Yes

Performed By:	Date:
Verified By:	Date:

℞	**Computer Qualification Protocol**	Protocol No.: 5048

Title: (Any Computer Co.) Model 575 Computer	Page: 31 of 62

6.2   Control Functions (Continued.)

Item No.	Expected Results	Results	Acceptable (Yes/No)
MAIN MENU - Supervisor (Continued.)			
39	After selecting the Key Button, the Logon/Logoff Window is displayed.	AE	Yes
40	After selecting the arrow in the User Name box, (3) options are displayed: Administrator, Supervisor, and User.	AE	Yes
41	After selecting the OK Button, the selection is accepted.	AE	Yes
42	After selecting Cancel, the Product Labeling Manager screen is displayed.	AE	Yes
43	After selecting the (grayed out) Hand Button, nothing happens.	AE	Yes
44	After selecting the (grayed out) Pages Plus Arrow-Left Button, nothing happens.	AE	Yes
45	After selecting the (grayed out) Pages Plus Arrow-Right Button, nothing happens.	AE	Yes
46	After selecting the (grayed out) Rx Button, nothing happens.	AE	Yes
47	After selecting the (grayed out) X (Clear Buffer) Button, nothing happens.	AE	Yes
48	After selecting the (grayed out) Magnifying Glass, nothing happens.	AE	Yes

Performed By:		Date:
Verified By:		Date:

℞	**Computer Qualification Protocol**	Protocol No.: 5048

Title: (Any Computer Co.) Model 575 Computer	Page: 32 of 62

6.2 Control Functions (Continued.)

Item No.	Expected Results	Results	Acceptable (Yes/No)
MAIN MENU - Administrator			
1	After selecting Product Labeling Manager from the Start push-up menu, the main screen displays (8) Pull Down Menus: File, View, Tools (grayed out), Data (grayed out), Security, User (grayed out), Configure (grayed out), and Help. Also displayed are the (10) Buttons: Rx, Open Book, Open Calendar, Key, Hand (grayed out), Pages Plus Arrow-Left (grayed out), Pages Plus Arrow-Right (grayed out), Rx (grayed out), X (grayed out), and Magnifying Glass (grayed out). Also displayed is the Status Bar.	AE	Yes
2	After selecting the File Pull-Down Menu (1) option is displayed: Exit (grayed out).	AE	Yes
3	After selecting Exit, nothing happens.	AE	Yes
4	After selecting the View Pull-Down Menu (5) options are displayed: Toolbar (with a checkmark in front of it), Status Bar (with a checkmark in front of it), View Product Data, Job Status and Job History.	AE	Yes

Performed By:	Date:
Verified By:	Date:

℞ **Computer Qualification Protocol**		Protocol No.: 5048	
Title: (Any Computer Co.) Model 575 Computer			Page: 33 of 62

6.2   Control Functions (Continued.)

Item No.	Expected Results	Results	Acceptable (Yes/No)
MAIN MENU - Administrator (Continued.)			
5	After selecting Toolbar, the Toolbar disappears. After selecting Toolbar again, the Toolbar reappears.	AE	Yes
6	After selecting Status Bar, the Status Bar disappears. After selecting the Status Bar again the Status Bar reappears.	AE	Yes
7	After selecting View Product Data, the View Product Data Window is displayed and (1) button: Close.	AE	Yes
8	After Close is selected the Product Labeling Manager screen is displayed.	AE	Yes
9	After selecting Job Status, the Job Status window is displayed and (4) Buttons are displayed: Pause, Refresh, Start and Close.	AE	Yes
10	After selecting Pause, the window remains the same without updates allowing the user to scroll left and right without refreshing the screen.	AE	Yes
11	After selecting Refresh, the window will be updated.	AE	Yes
12	After selecting Start, the window will return to updating data at set intervals.	AE	Yes
Performed By:		Date:	
Verified By:		Date:	

R̸ Computer Qualification Protocol		Protocol No.: 5048	
Title: (Any Computer Co.) Model 575 Computer			Page: 34 of 62

6.2 Control Functions (Continued.)

Item No.	Expected Results	Results	Acceptable (Yes/No)
MAIN MENU - Administrator (Continued.)			
13	After selecting Close, the Product Labeling Manager Main screen is displayed.	AE	Yes
14	After selecting View Drop-Down Menu, the Job History window is displayed and (1) Button: Close.	AE	Yes
15	After selecting Close, the Product Labeling Manager screen is displayed.	AE	Yes
16	After selecting the (grayed out) Tools Drop-Down Menu, nothing happens.	AE	Yes
17	After selecting the Security Drop-Down Menu, (2) options are displayed: Logon/Logoff, Administer (grayed out).	AE	Yes
18	After selecting Logon/Logoff, the Logon/Logoff window is displayed and (2) Buttons: OK, Cancel.	AE	Yes
19	After selecting the arrow in the User Name box, (3) options are displayed: Administrator, Supervisor, and User.	AE	Yes
20	After selecting the OK Button, the selection is accepted.	AE	Yes
21	After selecting Cancel, the Product Labeling Manager screen is displayed.	AE	Yes
Performed By:		Date:	
Verified By:		Date:	

R̠ **Computer Qualification Protocol**		Protocol No.: 5048
Title: (Any Computer Co.) Model 575 Computer		Page: 35 of 62

6.2   **Control Functions** (Continued.)

Item No.	Expected Results	Results	Acceptable (Yes/No)
MAIN MENU - Administrator (Continued.)			
22	After selecting the (grayed out) User Pull-Down menu, nothing happens.	AE	Yes
23	After selecting the (grayed out) Configure Pull-Down menu, nothing happens.	AE	Yes
24	After selecting the Help Pull-Down Menu, (2) options are displayed: Contents and About.	AE	Yes
25	After selecting Contents, a secondary Drop-Down Menu is displayed with (2) options: Extract Help Files and View On-Line Help.	AE	Yes
26	After selecting Extract Help Files, the On-Line Help Window is displayed and (1) Button: OK.	AE	Yes
27	After selecting OK, the Product Labeling Manager screen is displayed.	AE	Yes
28	After selecting View, then View On-Line Help, the Frameset 1- Microsoft Internet Explorer Window with the Table of Contents for the Product Labeling Manager Program is displayed.	AE	Yes
29	After selecting the X Button in the upper right corner, the Product Labeling Manager screen is displayed.	AE	Yes

Performed By:	Date:
Verified By:	Date:

Ŗ Computer Qualification Protocol		Protocol No.: 5048	
Title: (Any Computer Co.) Model 575 Computer			Page: 36 of 62

6.2 Control Functions (Continued.)

Item No.	Expected Results	Results	Acceptable (Yes/No)
MAIN MENU - Administrator (Continued.)			
30	After selecting the Rx Button (Left side of screen), the Product Data Window is displayed and (1) Button: Close.	AE	Yes
31	After selecting the Close Button, the Product Labeling Manager screen is displayed.	AE	Yes
32	After selecting the Open Book Button, the Current Job Status Window is displayed.	AE	Yes
33	After selecting Pause, the window remains the same without updates allowing the user to scroll left and right without refreshing the screen.	AE	Yes
34	After selecting Refresh, the window will be updated.	AE	Yes
35	After selecting Start, the window will return to updating data at set intervals.	AE	Yes
36	After selecting Close, the Product Labeling Manager Main screen is displayed.	AE	Yes
37	After selecting Open Calendar Button, the Job History Window is displayed and (1) Button: Close.	AE	Yes
38	After selecting the Close Button, the Product Labeling Manager screen is displayed.	AE	Yes
Performed By:		Date:	
Verified By:		Date:	

R̞ **Computer Qualification Protocol**		Protocol No.: 5048	
Title: (Any Computer Co.) Model 575 Computer		Page: 37 of 62	

6.2 **Control Functions** (Continued.)

Item No.	Expected Results	Results	Acceptable (Yes/No)
MAIN MENU - Administrator (Continued.)			
39	After selecting the Key Button, the Logon/Logoff Window is displayed.	AE	Yes
40	After selecting the arrow in the User Name box, (3) options are displayed: Administrator, Supervisor, and User.	AE	Yes
41	After selecting the OK Button, the selection is accepted.	AE	Yes
42	After selecting Cancel, the Product Labeling Manager screen is displayed.	AE	Yes
43	After selecting the (grayed out) Hand Button, nothing happens.	AE	Yes
44	After selecting the (grayed out) Pages Plus Arrow-Left Button, nothing happens.	AE	Yes
45	After selecting the (grayed out) Pages Plus Arrow-Right Button, nothing happens.	AE	Yes
46	After selecting the (grayed out) Rx Button, nothing happens.	AE	Yes
47	After selecting the (grayed out) X (Clear Buffer) Button, nothing happens.	AE	Yes
48	After selecting the (grayed out) Magnifying Glass, nothing happens.	AE	Yes
Performed By:		Date:	
Verified By:		Date:	

℞ **Computer Qualification Protocol**		Protocol No.: 5048	
Title: (Any Computer Co.) Model 575 Computer			Page: 38 of 62

6.3   System Functionality

6.3.1   Log-On/Log-Off System Security

Objective. To verify the three level password security system (Administrator, Supervisor and User) only allows access to the level assigned by the password. In the Results column, specify "AE" for "as expected" or if not enter information.

Item No.	Expected Results	Results	Acceptable (Yes/No)
Administrator Log-On Privileges			
1	After selecting the Key Button, the logon/logoff window is displayed.	AE	Yes
2	After selecting the User Name Entry Field drop down arrow, three options are displayed: Administrator, Supervisor and User.	AE	Yes
3	After selecting Administrator, the word Administrator is displayed in the User Name Entry Field.	AE	Yes
4	After entering 111111 in the Password Entry Field and clicking the OK button, the Product Labeling Manager main screen is displayed and none of the drop down menu options or buttons is grayed out.	AE	Yes
5	After selecting the Key Button, the Logon/Logoff window is displayed and the User Name Entry Field drop down arrow is grayed out.	AE	Yes

Performed By:		Date:
Verified By:		Date:

Ɍ **Computer Qualification Protocol**	Protocol No.: 5048

Title: (Any Computer Co.) Model 575 Computer	Page: 39 of 62

6.3.1   Log-On/Log-Off System Security (Continued.)

Item No.	Expected Results	Results	Acceptable (Yes/No)
6	After selecting the Cancel Button, the Product Labeling Manager main screen reappears and is unchanged from step 4.	AE	Yes
7	After selecting the Security drop down option and clicking on Logon/Logoff in the drop down menu, the Logon/Logoff window is displayed and the User Name Entry Field drop down arrow is grayed out.	AE	Yes
8	After selecting the Logoff Button, the Product Labeling Manager main screen is displayed with Tools, Data, User, Configure drop down menu options and the Hand, Pages plus left arrow, Pages plus right arrow, Rx, X, and Magnifying Glass icons are grayed out.	AE	Yes
9	After selecting the Key Button and Administrator from the User Name Entry Field drop down list, enter 222222 in the Password Entry Field then click the OK Button, the Logon Error message is displayed, stating Invalid Username/Password entry.	AE	Yes
10	After selecting the OK Button in the Logon Error window, the Logon/Logoff window is displayed.	AE	Yes

Performed By:	Date:
Verified By:	Date:

R **Computer Qualification Protocol**	Protocol No.: 5048

Title: (Any Computer Co.) Model 575 Computer	Page: 40 of 62

6.3.1   Log-On/Log-Off System Security (Continued.)

Item No.	Expected Results	Results	Acceptable (Yes/No)
11	After selecting Administrator from the User Name Entry Field drop down list, enter 333333 in the Password Entry Field, then select the OK Button, the Logon Error message is displayed, stating Invalid Username/Password entry.	AE	Yes
12	After selecting the OK Button in the Logon Error window, the Logon/Logoff window is displayed.	AE	Yes
13	After selecting Supervisor from the User Name Entry Field drop down list, enter 222222 in the Password Entry Field then select the OK button, the Product Labeling Manager main screen appears with Tools and the Hand Buttons grayed out, and Supervisor appears as a drop down menu option.	AE	Yes
14	After selecting Logon/Logoff from the Security drop down menu, the Logon/Logoff window is displayed. Next select the Logoff button, the Product Labeling Manager main screen appears with Tools, Data, User, Configure drop down menu options and the Hand, Pages plus left arrow, Pages plus right arrow, Rx, X, and Magnifying Glass Buttons are grayed out.	AE	Yes
15	After selecting the Key Button and Supervisor from the User Name Entry Field drop down list, enter 111111 in the Password Entry Field then select the OK button, the Logon Error message is displayed stating Invalid Username/Password entry.	AE	Yes

Performed By:	Date:
Verified By:	Date:

R **Computer Qualification Protocol**		Protocol No.: 5048
Title: (Any Computer Co.) Model 575 Computer		Page: 41 of 62

6.3.1   **Log-On/Log-Off System Security** (Continued.)

Item No.	Expected Results	Results	Acceptable (Yes/No)
16	After selecting the OK Button in the Logon Error window, the Logon/Logoff window is displayed.	AE	Yes
17	After selecting Supervisor from the User Name Entry Field drop down list, enter 333333 in the Password Entry Field then select the OK Button, the Logon Error message appears stating "Invalid Username/Password entry."	AE	Yes
18	After selecting the OK Button in the Logon Error window, the Logon/Logoff window is displayed.	AE	Yes
19	After selecting User from the User Name Entry Field drop down list, enter 333333 in the Password Entry Field. Next select the OK Button, the Product Labeling Manager main screen appears with Tools, Configure, Hand, Pages plus Right Arrow Buttons (grayed out) and User displays a drop down menu option.	AE	Yes
20	After selecting the Key Button, the Logon/Logoff window is displayed with the User Name Entry Field drop down arrow grayed out.	AE	Yes
21	After selecting the Cancel Button, the Product Labeling Manager main screen reappears and is unchanged from step 19.	AE	Yes

Performed By:		Date:
Verified By:		Date:

Ŗ Computer Qualification Protocol		Protocol No.: 5048	
Title: (Any Computer Co.) Model 575 Computer			Page: 42 of 62

6.3.1 Log-On/Log-Off System Security (Continued.)

Item No.	Expected Results	Results	Acceptable (Yes/No)
22	After selecting the "Logoff" button, the Product Labeling Manager main screen is displayed with Tools, Data, User, Configure drop down menu options. Hand, Pages plus left arrow, Pages plus right arrow, Rx, X, and Magnifying Glass Buttons are grayed out.	AE	Yes
Administrators' Log-On Privileges			
23	After selecting the Security drop down menu, select logon/logoff from the drop down list or click on the Key Button. From the Logon/Logoff window, select the User Name Entry Field drop down arrow, choose Administrator, then enter 111111 in the Password Entry Field. Next click on the OK Button and the Product Labeling Manager main screen appears with no grayed out drop down menu options or buttons and Administrator is a menu option.	AE	Yes
24	After selecting Tools, the drop down menu is displayed and nothing is grayed out.	AE	Yes
25	After selecting Backup Database from the Tools drop down menu, the Backup/Restore database window is displayed.	AE	Yes
26	After selecting the Cancel Button, a confirming Backup/Restore Database window appears informing the user that "Database backup/Restore canceled."	AE	Yes
Performed By:		Date:	
Verified By:		Date:	

Rx **Computer Qualification Protocol**		Protocol No.: 5048
Title: (Any Computer Co.) Model 575 Computer		Page: 43 of 62

6.3.1   **Log-On/Log-Off System Security** (Continued.)

Item No.	Expected Results	Results	Acceptable (Yes/No)
27	After selecting the OK Button, the Product Labeling Manager main window appears.	AE	Yes
28	After selecting Tools, Backup Database, and OK in the Backup/Restore Database window stops the Data Monitor and the Data Monitor window appears.	AE	Yes
29	After selecting the No Button, the Backup/Restore Database confirming window appears informing the user that "Database backup/restore canceled…"	AE	Yes
30	After selecting the Yes Button in the Data Monitor window, the database is backup and the Backup/Restore Database window is displayed with the message "Database backup successful."	AE	Yes
31	After selecting the Cancel Button in the Backup/Restore Database window, a warning note appears in the Backup/Restore Database window stating "Data Monitor was not started."	AE	Yes
32	After selecting the OK Button, the Product Labeling Manager's main window is displayed.	AE	Yes
33	When you select Data Monitoring from the Tools menu, the Data Monitor window is displayed. The traffic light shows red and states "Stopped."	AE	Yes

Performed By:	Date:
Verified By:	Date:

Ŗ̃ Computer Qualification Protocol		Protocol No.: 5048	
Title: (Any Computer Co.) Model 575 Computer			Page: 44 of 62

6.3.1 Log-On/Log-Off System Security (Continued.)

Item No.	Expected Results	Results	Acceptable (Yes/No)
34	After selecting the Start Button, if no lines are currently running, a small Data Monitor window appears stating "No Active Lines...Nothing to do!"	AE	Yes
35	After selecting the OK Button, the original Data Monitor window is displayed.	AE	Yes
36	After placing the cursor on the pointer and moving it, the frequency of monitoring is adjusted.	AE	Yes
37	After selecting the Expand Button, a drop down view of the Status window is displayed.	AE	Yes
38	After selecting the Close Button, the Product Labeling Manager's main window is displayed.	AE	Yes
39	After selecting Tools, Restore Database in the Backup/Restore Database the database window is displayed.	AE	Yes
40	After selecting Tools, Compact Database, the Compact Database window is displayed.	AE	Yes
41	After selecting the Cancel Button, the Compact Database message window appears stating "Database compaction canceled..."	AE	Yes
42	After selecting the OK Button in the Compact Database message window, the Product Labeling Manager main window is displayed.	AE	Yes

Performed By:	Date:
Verified By:	Date:

₨ **Computer Qualification Protocol**		Protocol No.: 5048

Title: (Any Computer Co.) Model 575 Computer	Page: 45 of 62

6.3.1   Log-On/Log-Off System Security (Continued.)

Item No.	Expected Results	Results	Acceptable (Yes/No)
43	After selecting the OK Button in the Compact Database window, the Data Monitor window message is displayed.	AE	Yes
44	After selecting No in the Data Monitor message window, the Compact Database message window appears stating "Database compaction canceled..."	AE	Yes
45	After selecting the OK Button in the Compact Database message window, the Product Labeling Manager main window is displayed.	AE	Yes
46	After selecting Tools, Manage History, the Manage History Data window is displayed.	AE	Yes
47	After highlighting any field, you are able to delete and enter new information.	AE	Yes
48	After selecting Data, Import Data from the drop down menu, the Import Data window is displayed.	AE	Yes
49	After selecting a Folder from the C drive list and a file from the files listed and selecting OK, the Import Data Confirm window is displayed.	AE	Yes
50	After selecting OK, the Import Data confirm window appears stating "Import was successful."	AE	Yes
51	After selecting OK again, the Product Labeling Manager main window is displayed.	AE	Yes

Performed By:		Date:
Verified By:		Date:

R Computer Qualification Protocol		Protocol No.: 5048
Title: (Any Computer Co.) Model 575 Computer		Page: 46 of 62

6.3.1 Log-On/Log-Off System Security (Continued.)

Item No.	Expected Results	Results	Acceptable (Yes/No)
52	After selecting Data Export, the Data Export window is displayed.	AE	Yes
53	After selecting Security, Administer, the User Administration window is displayed.	AE	Yes
54	After selecting Administrator and Products, the Select a Product Window is displayed.	AE	Yes
55	After selecting Administrator, Clear Buffer from the drop down menu, the Packaging Line Buffer Editor window is displayed.	AE	Yes
56	After selecting Administrator, Reports, the Reports selection window is displayed.	AE	Yes
57	After selecting Configure, Program Drive/Paths, the Program Properties window is displayed.	AE	Yes
58	After selecting the Hand Button, the User Administration window is displayed.	AE	Yes
59	After selecting the Pages Plus Left Arrow Icon, the Import Data window is displayed.	AE	Yes
60	After selecting the Pages Plus Right Arrow Icon, the Export Data window is displayed.	AE	Yes
61	After selecting the second Rx Icon, the Select a Product window is displayed.	AE	Yes
Performed By:		Date:
Verified By:		Date:

R Computer Qualification Protocol			Protocol No.: 5048

Title: (Any Computer Co.) Model 575 Computer	Page: 47 of 62

6.3.1 Log-On/Log-Off System Security (Continued.)

Item No.	Expected Results	Results	Acceptable (Yes/No)
62	After selecting the X Button, the Packaging Line Buffer Editor window is displayed.	AE	Yes
63	After selecting the Magnifying Glass Button, the Reports window is displayed.	AE	Yes
Supervisor Log-On Privileges			
64	After logging on as a supervisor, the Tools drop down menu is grayed out.	AE	Yes
65	After selecting Supervisor, Products, Clear Buffer and Reports, they are all available and they operate the same as the Administrator #23, except Security and Administrator are grayed out. Also the Hand Button is grayed out.	AE	Yes
User Log-On Privileges			
66	After selecting User, the Tools, Configure drop down menus are grayed out and (File, Exit), (Security, Administrator), (Data and Export) are grayed out. Also, the following Buttons are grayed out: Hand, Pages Plus Right Arrow. Every thing else operates the same as the Supervisor #65.	AE	Yes
67	After selecting View, View Product Data, the View Product Data window is read only.	AE	Yes

Performed By:	Date:
Verified By:	Date:

Ŗ Computer Qualification Protocol	Protocol No.: 5048	
Title: (Any Computer Co.) Model 575 Computer		Page: 48 of 62

6.3.2   Importing Product Data

Objective. To verify the computer system is able to import data into the import data file without any system errors. In the Results column, specify "AE" for "as expected" or if not enter information.

Item No.	Expected Results	Results	Acceptable (Yes/No)
Administrator, Supervisor and User			
1	After selecting Data then Import Data from the pull-down menu, the Import Data window is displayed.	AE	Yes
2	After selecting the appropriate drive from the Drives drop down list, the Import Data window is displayed.	AE	Yes
3	After selecting the Import Data file from the Folders file list the Import Data file is displayed.	AE	Yes
4	After selecting the Import Data filename from the Files list box, the import test box is displayed.	AE	Yes
5	After selecting the OK Button, the importing process is completed. Verify that the data was imported.	AE	Yes
6	After selecting Cancel, the Import Data window is displayed.	AE	Yes

Performed By:	Date:
Verified By:	Date:

R **Computer Qualification Protocol**	Protocol No.: 5048
Title: (Any Computer Co.) Model 575 Computer	Page: 49 of 62

6.3.3   Exporting Product Data

Objective. To verify the Case Labeling System is able to export data to a designated drive and folder without any system errors. In the Results column, specify "AE" for "as expected" or if not enter information.

Item No.	Expected Results	Results	Acceptable (Yes/No)
Administrator, Supervisor and User			
1	After selecting Data Export Data Export window is displayed.	AE	Yes
2	After selecting All or Partial from the Export Data window and the export filter Type from the Type drop-down menu, then enter the required information into the Item No., Begin Date and End date text boxes; select the Drive and Folder to export to; enter the file name in the Export Filename text box, then select the OK Button, the exporting process is completed.	AE	Yes
3	After selecting Cancel, the export Data window is displayed.	AE	Yes

Performed By:	Date:
Verified By:	Date:

℞	**Computer Qualification Protocol**	Protocol No.: 5048

Title: (Any Computer Co.) Model 575 Computer	Page: 50 of 62

6.3.4 Managing Product Data

Objective. To verify that new data can be added to the Product Data File and existing data can be modified. In the Results column, specify "AE" for "as expected" or if not enter information.

Item No.	Expected Results	Results	Acceptable (Yes/No)
Administrator and Supervisor			
1	After selecting View Product Data from the View pull down menu, the View Product Data window is displayed.	AE	Yes
2	After scrolling to the bottom of the Product List, enter new product data, select Close, next select View Product Data to verify that the new data was recorded.	AE	Yes
3	After scrolling to the desired product position the cursor in the desired field and make a change. Next select Close. Then select View Product Data to verify that the data was changed.	AE	Yes
4	After scrolling to the desired product, highlight the product record by selecting the selector button left of the Item Number field then press the delete Key and select Close. Next select View Product Data to verify that the data was deleted.	AE	Yes

Performed By:	Date:
Verified By:	Date:

℞ **Computer Qualification Protocol**	Protocol No.: 5048
Title: (Any Computer Co.) Model 575 Computer	Page: 51 of 62

6.3.5   Managing History Data

Objective. To verify that new data can be added to the History of a product and existing data can be modified. In the Results column, specify "AE" for "as expected" or if not enter information.

Item No.	Expected Results	Results	Acceptable (Yes/No)
Administrator			
1	After selecting View Product History Data from the View pull down menu, the View Product Data window is displayed.	AE	Yes
2	After scrolling to the desired product position the cursor in the desired field and make a change. Next select Close. Then select View Product History Data to verify that the data was changed.	AE	Yes
3	After scrolling to the desired product, highlight the product record by selecting the selector button left of the Item Number field then press the delete Key and select Close. Next select View Product History Data to verify that the data was deleted.	AE	Yes

Performed By:	Date:
Verified By:	Date:

℞ **Computer Qualification Protocol**	Protocol No.: 5048
Title: (Any Computer Co.) Model 575 Computer	Page: 52 of 62

6.3.6 View the Current Job Status

Objective. To verify that the current status of the labeling jobs running on the packaging lines can be viewed. In the Results column, specify "AE" for "as expected" or if not enter information.

Item No.	Expected Results	Results	Acceptable (Yes/No)
All Users			
1	After selecting the Open Book Button, the Current Job Status window is displayed.	AE	Yes
2	After selecting the Pause Button to pause the refresh rate of the dialog, use the right/left scroll controls to scroll through the available data then select the Refresh Button to view the up-to-date data from the Qty Verified and QtyNoReadMatch fields.	AE	Yes
3	Select the Close Button to close the job status dialog.	AE	Yes

Performed By:	Date:
Verified By:	Date:

R **Computer Qualification Protocol**			Protocol No.: 5048	
Title: (Any Computer Co.) Model 575 Computer				Page: 53 of 62

6.3.7 Starting a Labeling Job

Objective. To verify that a labeling job can be started. In the Results column, specify "AE" for "as expected" or if not enter information.

Item No.	Expected Results	Results	Acceptable (Yes/No)
1	After selecting the Product from the Administrator Window, the Products window is displayed.	AE	Yes
2	After selecting an Item Number from the drop down list and a Case Size from the Case Size drop down list, enter a Batch number into the Batch Number text box, Quantity, Expiration Date, Packaging Line, then select OK. The following dialog is presented to verify the previously entered data: Product Description; Product Number; Item Number; Batch Number; Expiration Date; Case Size, Quantity and Packaging Size.	AE	Yes
3	After selecting the Override Button, data can be corrected/modified.	AE	Yes
4	After selecting the OK Button a test label is generated and the following message box is provided: Packaging Line; Product Desc; Item Number; Batch Number; Case Number; Expiration Date and Number of Labels.	AE	Yes

Performed By:			Date:
Verified By:			Date:

R	**Computer Qualification Protocol**	Protocol No.: 5048
Title: (Any Computer Co.) Model 575 Computer		Page: 54 of 62

6.3.7 **Starting a Labeling Job** (Continued.)

Item No.	Expected Results	Results	Acceptable (Yes/No)
5	After selecting the OK Button, the following appears: The packaging line decoder will be reset; the packaging line decoder will be configured; the labeling job will be transmitted to the packaging line printer; the software will return control to the Product dialog. After selecting the Close Button the Product dialog window will close.	AE	Yes
6	After selecting the Cancel Button, the Product Labeling manager window is displayed.	AE	Yes

Performed By:	Date:
Verified By:	Date:

℞ **Computer Qualification Protocol**	Protocol No.: 5048
Title: (Any Computer Co.) Model 575 Computer	Page: 55 of 62

6.3.8   Using the Data Monitor

Objective. To verify that the data monitor for all packaging lines which are configured with active packaging jobs can be manually started and stopped. Also, to verify that the administrator can view the communications with the decoders as updated information is retrieved. In the Results column, specify "AE" for "as expected" or if not enter information.

Item No.	Expected Results	Results	Acceptable (Yes/No)
Administrator			
1	After selecting the Tools Menu, the Data Monitor window is displayed.	AE	Yes
2	After selecting the Start Button, the data monitor function for all active packaging lines is started.	AE	Yes
3	After selecting the Stop Button, the data monitor function for all active packaging lines is stopped.	AE	Yes
4	After selecting the Contract/Expand Button, data monitor dialog can be sized.	AE	Yes
5	After selecting Close, the data monitor is closed.	AE	Yes

Performed By:	Date:
Verified By:	Date:

℞ **Computer Qualification Protocol**	Protocol No.: 5048
Title: (Any Computer Co.) Model 575 Computer	Page: 56 of 62

6.3.9 Creating Reports

Objective. To verify that reports can be created. In the Results column, specify "AE" for "as expected" or if not enter information.

Note: This function is not being used at this time. If there is ever a requirement for this function in the future, it will be validated at that time and added to the protocol with an addendum.

Item No.	Expected Results	Results	Acceptable (Yes/No)
	None.		

Performed By:	Date:
Verified By:	Date:

℞ **Computer Qualification Protocol**	Protocol No.: 5048
Title: (Any Computer Co.) Model 575 Computer	Page: 57 of 62

6.3.10   Retention of Data After Loss of Power

Objective. To document data retention by the Case Labeling System after experiencing a loss of power.

Procedure

1. Start the print and apply system.
2. Enter the necessary information to begin printing labels at an available packaging line. Verify the print job has been sent to the packaging line from the Data Monitor screen.
3. Begin entering the information for printing labels at a second packaging line.
4. Before accepting the print job to be sent to the line, turn the PC off.
5. Wait thirty seconds, and restart the Case Labeling System.
6. Document any procedures necessary to restore the print and apply system to its original state prior to the loss of power in the results section.
7. Verify that the information for the second print job must be re-entered and that the first print job entered is tracking and printing labels with no interruptions.

Expected Results	Results	Acceptable (Yes/No)
After restoring power, the Case Labeling System starts.	AE	Yes
The first print job entered is displayed under the appropriate packaging line on the Data Monitor screen. The print job continues to track and print labels without interruption.	AE	Yes
The information for the second print job is missing and must be re-entered.	AE	Yes

Performed By:	Date:
Verified By:	Date:

R̟ **Computer Qualification Protocol**	Protocol No.: 5048
Title: (Any Computer Co.) Model 575 Computer	Page: 58 of 62

7.0 Performance Qualification (PQ)

Once it has been established that the Computer system is properly installed and functioning within specified operating parameters, it must be shown that the computer system can be operated reliably under routine operating conditions.

7.1 Computer System Operation

Test Objective. The objective of the test is to verify the performance of the Case Labeling Septum on packaging line 1 by observing the system in normal production operation.

Test Procedure

- Observe at least 2 packaging runs consisting of approximately 30 cases on packaging line 1, documenting all parameters listed below. Verify that the print and apply system performs as it is intended without causing a disruption to the packaging process. Record the results in Tables XII and XIII.

- Include copies of each production Report generated by the print and apply system at the completion of each packaging run, in Attachment 2.

Acceptance Criteria

The print and apply septum on packaging line 1 performs as it is intended to and does not cause any disruption affecting the performance of packaging line 1 as a complete system. Note: the number of conveyor belt stops is for information only.

Prepared By:	Date:
Verified By:	Date:

Rᵪ **Computer Qualification Protocol**			Protocol No.: 5048	
Title: (Any Computer Co.) Model 575 Computer				Page: 59 of 62

Table XII   Test Results

First Packaging Run Observed		
Number of Conveyor Belt Stops		**Results**
Conveyor belt stops for unacceptable case labels		AE
Print and Apply System performs without disruptions		AE
Performance		**Acceptable (Yes/No)**
Print and Apply System performs without disruptions		Yes
Parameters		
Product Name: Any product	Batch Number: 73419	Case Size:
Number of Cases: 100	Date: 07/23/98	Total Time: 30 Min.

Prepared By:	Date:
Verified By:	Date:

℞ **Computer Qualification Protocol**	Protocol No.: 5048
Title: (Any Computer Co.) Model 575 Computer	Page: 60 of 62

Table XIII Test Results

Second Packaging Run Observed	
Number of Conveyor Belt Stops	**Results**
Conveyor belt stops for unacceptable case labels	AE
Print and Apply System performs without disruptions	AE
Performance	**Acceptable (Yes/No)**
Print and Apply System performs without disruptions	Yes
Parameters		

Product Name: Any product	Batch Number: 73420	Case Size:
Number of Cases: 100	Date: 07/23/98	Total Time: 29 Min.

Prepared By:	Date:
Verified By:	Date:

℞ **Computer Qualification Protocol**	Protocol No.: 5048
Title: (Any Computer Co.) Model 575 Computer	Page: 61 of 62

Attachment 1

Hard Drive Directory Listings

R **Computer Qualification Protocol**	Protocol No.: 5048
Title: (Any Computer Co.) Model 575 Computer	Page: 62 of 62

Attachment 2

Production Reports

Appendix F

Process Qualification Protocol Example

I have included an actual qualification protocol template that is filled in to show you an example of how to develop a process qualification protocol. Each of the protocol elements is covered in the template. Note that process qualification protocols do not follow the usual IQ, OQ, and PQ format; they contain only a PQ.

R̥	**Process Qualification Protocol**	
Title: (Product Name) Tablets USP 300/30 mg		Protocol No.: 7156
Process/Formula: 10/10		Page: 1 of 18
Batch Size: 2,500,000 Units	Catalog Number: 2571	
Prepared By:		
Validation:		Date:
Approved By:		
Validation Manager:		Date:
Research & Development:		Date:
Operations:		Date:
Maintenance:		Date:
Regulatory Compliance:		Date:

Ŗ	**Process Qualification Protocol**	Protocol No.: 7156
Title: (Product Name) Tablets USP 300/30 mg		Page: 2 of 18

1.0 Table of Contents

R̥	**Process Qualification Protocol**	Protocol No.: 7156
Title: (Product Name) Tablets USP 300/30 mg		Page: 3 of 18

2.0   Objective

To establish documented evidence which provides a high degree of assurance that this specific process will consistently produce (Product Name) tablets USP 300/30 mg, meeting predetermined acceptance criteria and quality attributes by performing the following tests.

2.1   Test Function Definitions

1   Raw Material Characterization
2   Blend Analysis
3   Bulk Density, Tapped Density and Angle of Repose Analysis
4   Physical Analysis of the Compression Process
5   Content Uniformity
6   Finished Product Analysis
7   Dissolution Profile Comparison to Bio-Equivalency Batch

3.0   Scope

This protocol applies to the manufacture of (Product Name) Tablets USP 300/30 mg, Catalog No. 2571, Process/Formula 12/12, Batch Size 2,500,000 Units. Three connective batches will be manufactured by the Batch Record. Each batch must meet acceptance criteria specified in the above mentioned Test Functions 1 through 7. If any batch(es) fails due to process extrinsic causes or deviations from the Batch Record due to process extrinsic reasons, that batch(s) will be disqualified and an additional batch(es) will be manufactured to replace the deviated batch(es).

4.0   Process Description

(Product Name) Tablets USP 300/30 mg are first manufactured by weighing product ingredients then blending them in a 2123 liter twinshell blender. Approximately 15 kg of premixed ingredients and magnesium sterate are mixed in a polyethylene bag and passed through a 20 mesh screen. The remainder of the blend and the screened blend will be blended in a 2123 liter twinshell blender. The final blend is compressed using a Manesty Unipress, 34 station Press.

R̸ **Process Qualification Protocol**		Protocol No.: 7156	
Title: (Product Name) Tablets 300/30 mg			Page: 4 of 18

5.0   Unit and Batch Formula

Code No.	Ingredient	Amount Per Tablet	Quantity Per Batch
1603	(Any Chemical) Active	-	492.50 kg
-	(Any Chemical) USP	150.311 mg	-
-	(Any Chemical) USP	30.141 mg	-
-	Pregelatinized Starch NF	16.548 mg	-
1861	(Any Chemical) Active	-	416.75 kg
-	(Any Chemical) USP	150.030 mg	-
-	Pregelatinized Starch NF, Povidone USE, Crospovidone	16.670 mg	-
4202	Microcrystalline Cellulose NF	64.400 mg	161.00 kg
4712	Croscarmellose Sodium NF	9.000 mg	22.50 kg
7302	Sodium Lauryl Sulfate NF	0.900 mg	2,250 g
5302	Magnesium Sterate NF	2.250 mg	5,625 g
6002	Stearic Acid NF	3.500 mg	8,750 g
	Total Tablet Weight	443.750 mg	-

5.1 Major Equipment Used

2123 Liter Twinshell Blender, Equipment No. 453

Manesty Unipress 34 Station Press, Equipment No. 6411

Performed By:	Date:
Verified By:	Date:

℞	**Process Qualification Protocol**	Protocol No.: 7156

Title: (Product Name) Tablets 300/30 mg	Page: 5 of 18

5.2   Required Documentation

Record the standard operating procedures used to process the product in Table I.

Table I   Standard Operating Procedures

Number	Description	Release Date
DEV025	Validation Sampling	10/23/97
DEV026	Validation Department - Moisture Content Determination	03/12/96
DEV027	Operation of Ohaus Moisture Balances	10/23/97
DEV028	Blending and Granulation - Wet Granulation	03/12/96
DEV029	Blending and Granulation - Milling	10/23/97
DEV030	Verification/Determination of Unit Blend sample Chamber	03/12/96
DEV031	Blend Uniformity Acceptance Criteria	10/23/97
DEV032	Determination of Bulk Density, tapped Density and Angle of Repose	03/12/96
DEV033	Friability Testing	10/23/97
DEV034	Statistical Process Control for Compression	03/12/96
DEV035	Operations Acceptable Quality level Testing	10/23/97
DEV036	Determination of Individual Tablet Thickness	03/12/96
DEV037	Investigation Procedure	10/23/97
DEV038	Tablet Press Qualification	03/12/96

Performed By:	Date:
Verified By:	Date:

R **Process Qualification Protocol**	Protocol No.: 7156
Title: (Product Name) Tablets 300/30 mg	Page: 6 of 18

6.0 Test Functions

Test Function 1 - Raw Material Characterization

Objective. To verify that the active raw materials used in the validation batches and in the bio-equivalency batch meet their respective predetermined specifications.

Parameter	Method	Specification
Foreign Matter	MR-32	None Observed
Description	MR-1603	Meets Specification
(Any Chemical)	MR-1603	I.D. Positive
(Any Chemical)	MR-1603	I.D. Positive
Water	MR-1603	NMT 2.0%
(Any Chemical)	Cd No. 561	NMT 0.5%
(Any Chemical)	MR-1603	14.8 to 15.7%
Acetaminophen	MR-1603	74.4 to 78.2%
Starch ID	MR-1603	I.D. Positive
Heavy Metals	MR-1603	NMT 0.001%
Microbial Limits	MR-1603	-
Total Plate Count	-	NMT 1000/g
Yeast and Mold Count	-	NMT 100/g
Salmonella	-	Negative

Performed By:	Date:
Verified By:	Date:

R Process Qualification Protocol		Protocol No.: 7156
Title: (Product Name) Tablets 300/30 mg		Page: 7 of 18

Test Function 1 - Raw Material Characterization (Continued.)

Parameter	Method	Specification
E. Coli	-	Negative
Reserve Sample	MR-2	Completed
Manufacturer's Check	MR-5	Mallinckrodt
Description	MR-1861	Meets Specification
Identification	MR-1861	I.D. Positive
Starch ID	MR-1861	I.D. Positive
Water	MR-1603	0.6 to 1.5%
Assay	MR-1603	87.5 to 92.5%
Particle Size (Target)	MR-1603	25% Maximum Retained on 60 Mesh 75% Minimum Retained on 200 Mesh Cumulative
Degradation Products	CD-165	NMT 0.05%
Heavy Metals	MR-1861	NMT 0.001%
Microbial Limits:	MR-1861	-
Total Plate Count	-	NMT 1000/g
Yeast and Mold Count	-	NMT 100/g
Salmonella	-	Negative
E. Coli	-	Negative
Reserve Sample Preparation	MR-2	Completed
Performed By:		Date:
Verified By:		Date:

Ŗ **Process Qualification Protocol**	Protocol No.: 7156	
Title: (Product Name) Tablets 300/30 mg		Page: 8 of 18

Test Function 1 - Raw Material Characterization (Continued.)

Parameter	Method	Specification
Manufacturer's Check	MR-5	Mallinckrodt
Foreign Matter	MR-5	Mallinckrodt
Description	MR-1861	Meets Specification
Identification	MR-1861	I.D. Positive
Starch ID	MR-1861	I.D. Positive
Water	MR-1603	0.6 to 1.5%
Assay	MR-1603	87.5 to 92.5%
Particle Size (Target)	MR-1603	25% Maximum Retained on 60 Mesh 75% Minimum Retained on 200 Mesh Cumulative
Degradation Products	CD-165	NMT 0.05%
Heavy Metals	MR-1861	NMT 0.001%
Microbial Limits:	MR-1861	-
Total Plate Count	-	NMT 1000/g
Yeast and Mold Count	-	NMT 100/g
Salmonella	-	Negative
E. Coli	-	Negative
Reserve Sample Preparation	MR-2	Completed
Performed By:		Date:
Verified By:		Date:

℞	**Process Qualification Protocol**	Protocol No.: 7156

Title: (Product Name) Tablets USP 300/30 mg	Page: 9 of 18

Test Function 2 - Blend Analysis

Objective. To determine that there is uniform distribution of the active ingredient throughout the blend.

Acetaminophen 300 mg				
Batch No.	**Average$_{10}$**	**Range**	**RSD**	**Specification**
04267	101.3%	99.9-105.9%	2.0%	85.0% ≤ LSTL ≤ 115.0%
14267	99.2%	96.0-109.0%	4.0%	85.0% ≤ LSTL ≤ 115.0%
24267	100.5%	98.2-104.6%	2.2%	RSD ≤ 6.0%

Codeine 30 mg				
Batch No.	**Average$_{10}$**	**Range**	**RSD**	**Specification**
04267	104.5%	99.5-108.2%	2.8%	85.0% ≤ LSTL ≤ 115.0%
14267	104.2%	98.6-113.2%	3.9%	85.0% ≤ LSTL ≤ 115.0%
24267	100.3%	95.1-105.2%	3.9%	RSD ≤ 6.0%

Performed By:	Date:
Verified By:	Date:

R	**Process Qualification Protocol**	Protocol No.: 7156
Title: (Product Name) Tablets USP 300/30 mg		Page: 10 of 18

Test Function 3 - Bulk Density, Tapped Density and Angle of Repose Analysis

Objective. To determine the physical properties of the blend.

Batch No.	Bulk Density	Tapped Density	Angle of Repose	Acceptance Criteria
04267	0.541 g/ml	0.612 g/ml	38.6°	For informational
14267	0.533 g/ml	0.614 g/ml	38.3°	purposes only.
24267	0.529 g/ml	0.610 g/ml	38.8°	

Performed By:	Date:
Verified By:	Date:

℞	**Process Qualification Protocol**	Protocol No.: 7156
Title: (Product Name) Tablets USP 300/30 mg		Page: 11 of 18

Test Function 4 - Physical Analysis of the Compression Process

Objective. To verify that the compression process conforms to specifications and process capability.

Acceptance Criteria:

Target Weight: Target 10 = 4.44 g ±2.5%

Average Tablet Hardness: Target 12±4 Sc

Cpk = NLT 0.9

Tablet Press Speed: For informational purposes only.

Defects: Acceptable Quality Level

Procedure:

A process capability study will be performed on the data collected for weight and hardness testing per batch record for each tablet press used during compression. The data will be compared to the acceptance criteria to derive the Cpk.

An additional batch will be manufactured for informational purposes only to characterize the tableting speed and collect data for weight and hardness.   Compress the batch on as many presses as feasible. Document the tablet press speed at the slowest speed that the equipment will operate while making acceptable tablets on each tablet press involved. Run at the slow speed for approximately one hour. Document the tablet press speed at the fastest speed that the equipment will operate while making acceptable tablets on each tablet press used. Run at the fast speed for a minimum of one hour. Record the information in Tables II, III , IV and V.

℞ **Process Qualification Protocol**		Protocol No.: 7156	
Title: (Product Name) Tablets USP 300/30 mg			Page: 12 of 18

Test Function 4 - Physical Analysis of the Compression Process (Continued.)

Table II Acceptable Quality level Acetaminophen and Codeine 300/30 mg

Defects	04267	14267	24267
Critical (0)			
1. Foreign Product	0	0	0
Major A (NMT 2)			
1. Tablet not free of capping, cavitation or lamination.	0	0	0
Major B (NMT 21)			
1. Tablet not uniform in size, shape or color.	0	0	0
2. Tablet not free of major embedded surface spots.	0	0	0
3. Tablet not free of breaks or splits.	0	0	0
4. Debossing illegible.	0	0	0
5. Tablet not free of major sticking.	0	0	0
6. Tablet not free of major overturned or feathered edge.	0	0	0
Minor (NMT 21)			
1. Tablet not free of minor overturned or feathered edge.	0	0	0
2. Tablet not free of minor sticking.	0	0	0
3. Tablet not free of chips.	0	0	0
4. Debossing or crease not sharp.	0	0	0
5. Tablet not free of minor embedded surface spots.	0	0	0
Performed By:		Date:	
Verified By:		Date:	

R̶	**Process Qualification Protocol**		Protocol No.: 7156
Title: (Product Name) Tablets USP 300/30 mg			Page: 13 of 18

Test Function 4 - Physical Analysis of the Compression Process (Continued.)

Table III Tablet Weight

Batch No.	Average	Range	Acceptance Criteria
04267	4.459 g	4.370-4.550 g	Target Weight:
14267	4.427 g	4.370-4.470 g	10 = 4.44 g ±2.5%
24267	4.452 g	4.380-4.550 g	

Table IV Tablet Hardness

Batch No.	Average	Range	Acceptance Criteria
04267	13.340 Sc	11.000-15.500 Sc	Target Hardness:
14267	12.779 Sc	11.000-14.500 Sc	12 = ±4 Sc
24267	13.082 Sc	11.500-14.500 Sc	

Table V Tablet Press Speed

Batch No.	Slowest Speed	Fastest Speed	Acceptance Criteria
74258	51 rpm Total Time = 2 hrs	63 rpm Total Time = 1 hr	For informational purposes only.

Performed By:	Date:
Verified By:	Date:

R̶	**Process Qualification Protocol**	Protocol No.: 7156
Title: (Product Name) Tablets USP 300/30 mg		Page: 14 of 18

Test Function 5 - Content Uniformity

Objective. To verify product conformance to USP specifications

Acceptance Criteria:

APAP For 10 Tablets: 85.0-115.0%, RSD ≤6.0%

For 30 tablets, NMT 1 unit is outside the range of 85.0-115.0% and no unit is outside the range of 75.0-125.0, RSD ≤7.8%

Codeine For 10 Tablets: 85.0-115.0%, RSD ≤6.0%

For 30 tablets, NMT 1 unit is outside the range of 85.0-115.0% and no unit is outside the range of 75.0-125.0, RSD ≤7.8%

Procedure:

Adhere to the standard operating procedure, Validation Sampling (Content Uniformity). Record the results in Tables VI and VII.

R	**Process Qualification Protocol**			Protocol No.: 7156

Title: (Product Name) Tablets USP 300/30 mg	Page: 15 of 18

Test Function 5 - Content Uniformity (Continued.)

Table VI Acetaminophen 300 mg

Content Uniformity	Average	Range	RSD	Specification
04267 Beginning of Run Middle of Run End of Run	98.4% 102.2% 102.8%	94.2-100.7% 99.3-104.4% 99.4-105.7%	2.1% 1.7% 1.8%	For 10 tablets, 85.0-115.0%, RSD ≤6.0%

For 30 tablets, NMT |
| 04267 Beginning of Run Middle of Run End of Run | 96.7% 97.3% 99.1% | 91.8-103.3% 95.3-99.2% 91.2-105.4% | 3.2% 1.2% 3.4% | 1 unit is outside the range of 85.0-115.0%

No unit is outside the range of 75.0-125.0% |
| 04267 Beginning of Run Middle of Run End of Run | 97.6% 96.8% 99.3% | 91.8-105.5% 90.5-109.7% 96.5-102.5% | 3.6% 5.4% 2.4% | RSD ≤6.0% |

Performed By:	Date:
Verified By:	Date:

R	**Process Qualification Protocol**		Protocol No.: 7156
Title: (Product Name) Tablets USP 300/30 mg			Page: 16 of 18

Test Function 5 - Content Uniformity (Continued.)

Table VII Codeine 30 mg

Content Uniformity	Average	Range	RSD	Specification
04267 Beginning of Run Middle of Run End of Run	99.3% 104.9% 102.2%	96.8-101.4% 101.6-108.1% 100.3-104.2%	1.6% 1.7% 1.3%	For 10 tablets, 85.0-115.0%, RSD ≤6.0%
04267 Beginning of Run Middle of Run End of Run	97.5% 99.7% 103.1%	94.7-100.1% 92.8-104.5% 95.8-106.4%	1.9% 4.2% 2.9%	For 30 tablets, NMT 1 unit is outside the range of 85.0-115.0%
04267 Beginning of Run Middle of Run End of Run	100.7% 102.9% 101.9%	95.9-109.6% 100.5-107.7% 100.5-104.3%	5.2% 2.3% 1.6%	No unit is outside the range of 75.0-125.0% RSD ≤6.0%

Performed By:	Date:
Verified By:	Date:

R̥ **Process Qualification Protocol**	Protocol No.: 7156
Title: (Product Name) Tablets 300/30 mg	Page: 17 of 18

Test Function 6 - Finished Product Analysis

Objective. To verify that the finished product test results meet finished product specifications.

Parameter	Method	Specification
Description	CD-517	Conforms
(Any Chemical) 300.0 mg	USP XXII Supp. 3	90.0-110.0%
(Any Chemical) 30.0 mg	USP XXII Supp. 3	90.0-110.0%
Identification	USP XXII	I.D. Positive A and B
Dissolution: (Any Chemical)	USP XXII	NLT 75% in 45 Min.
Dissolution: (Any Chemical)	USP XXII	NLT 75% in 45 Min.
Uniformity of dosage units: (Any Chemical) Content uniformity	USP XXII Supp. 3	For 10 Tablets: 85.0-115.0%, RSD ≤6.0% For 30 tablets, 9 of 10: 85.0-115.0% RSD NMT 7.8%
Uniformity of dosage units: (Any Chemical) Content uniformity	USP XXII Supp. 3	For 10 Tablets: 85.0-115.0%, RSD ≤6.0% For 30 tablets, 9 of 10: 85.0-115.0% RSD NMT 7.8%

Performed By:	Date:
Verified By:	Date:

R	**Process Qualification Protocol**	Protocol No.: 7156
Title: (Product Name) Tablets USP 300/30 mg		Page: 18 of 18

Test Function 7 - Dissolution Profile Comparison to Bio-equivalency batch

Objective. To determine if the dissolution profiles for the validation batches are equivalent to the dissolution profile for the bio-equivalency batch.

Acceptance Criteria:

Dissolution to be NMT 75% (Q) in 45 Min.

The dissolution profile will be compared to the profile of the batch establishing bio-equivalency and will meet one or more of the following criteria based on a literature review of the product involved:

     a. Substantially matches at all points.

     b. Substantially matches at the most critical points based on the pharmacokinetics of the drug.

Procedure:

Adhere to the validation sampling (Dissolution).

Summary:

All three validation batches met Q of 75% in 45 minutes for both (Any Chemical) and (Any Chemical). They also displayed similar dissolution profiles to the lot submitted in the ANDA. The range of values at each dissolution time point was also similar. Based on these observations, the in vivo pharmacokinetics theoretically should be similar among these batches since the product is not known or suspected to have bio-equivalence problems.

Appendix G

Full-Size Lists and Forms

Equipment Master List

Protocol Master List

Project Status List

Document Master List

Document Database

Request for Validation Form

Document Review Form

Conditional Release Form

Certification Form

Validation Baseline Document

Validation Change Request Form

Deficiency Form

Protocol Package Contents Sheet

See Chapter 2 under "Equipment Master List" for information on how to develop and use an equipment master list.

℞	Equipment Master List			
Equipment Number	Serial Number	Description	Location/ Room	Reason Not Validated

See Chapter 2 under "Protocol Master List" for information on how to develop and use a protocol master list.

R̥	**Protocol Master List**					
Protocol Number	**Description**	**Equip. No.**	**Serial No.**	**Location /Room**	**Name**	**Com. Date**

See Chapter 4 under "Project Status List" for information on how to develop and use a project status list.

℞	Project Status List			
Protocol Number ⇨				

See Chapter 8 under "Document Master List" for information on how to develop and use a document master list.

℞ Document Master List				
Protocol Number ⇨				

See Chapter 9 under "Document Database" for information on how to develop and use a document database.

℞	Document Database					
Document Number	Description	Equip. No.	Serial No.	Location /Room	Name	Com. Date

See Chapter 2 under "Request for Validation Form" for information on how to develop and use a request for validation form.

R̸	**Request for Validation Form**	
Originator:	Date:	RFV No.:
Department:	Extension:	
Reason for Validation:		
Schedule Information:		
Equipment Name:	Manufacturer:	
Model Number:	Equipment Number:	
Serial Number:	Location:	
The following documentation shall be included with this request. (Check all that are included.) ❑ Capitol Appropriation Request ❑ Operations & Maintenance Manual ❑ Quote ❑ Drawings ❑ Purchase Order ❑ Operation & Cleaning SOPs (Can be in draft form) ❑ Invoice		
❑ Accept Testing to be conducted: IQ OQ PQ Priority: Routine Urgent Validation Specialist: Comments:	❑ Not Required (Explain.)	
Validation Manager Approval:	Date:	

Form Number: V001 (5/28/98)   Reference: SOP-VAL001

See Chapter 4 under "Document Review Form" for information on how to develop and use a document review form.

Ŗ̌	**Document Review Form**	
Originator:	Date:	DRF No.:

Document Number:
Title:

Documentation Types:

   ☐   Protocol   ☐   Requal Protocol   ☐   Final Report   ☐   Conditional Release Form

   ☐   Certification Form   ☐   Validation Baseline Document   ☐   Deficiency

   ☐   Addendum

Reviewer Response:

Select the appropriate option, then return your copy to validation. If no comments are received by (specified date) your concurrence will be assumed.

   ☐   Approved as is.

   ☐   Approved on condition that the attached comments are incorporated.

   ☐   Not approved, give reason.

Reviewer Signature:	Date:

Distribution:

   Research & Development
   Operations
   Maintenance
   Regulatory Compliance

Form Number: V002 (5/28/98)   Reference: SOP-VAL002

See Chapter 5 under "Conditional Release Form" for information on how to develop and use a conditional release form.

℞	**Conditional Release Form**		
Protocol Number: Title:		CRF No.:	
Manufacturer:			
Model Number:		Serial Number:	
Equipment Number:		Location:	

Statement

All of the qualification testing and verification is complete, therefore, the (system name) is released for use by (Department Name).

Conditional Release Date:

Originator:	Date:
Approved By: Validation Manager:	Date:

Form Number: V003 (5/28/98)   Reference: SOP-VAL003

See Chapter 5 under "System Certification Form" for information on how to develop and use a certification form.

℞	Certification Form	
Protocol No.: Title:		CF No.:
Manufacturer:		
Model Number:	Serial Number:	
Equipment Number:	Location:	
Statement Based upon the acceptable results of the qualification testing and any applicable follow-up actions, this (system name) has been found to meet all validation requirements defined herein.		
Originator:		Date:
Approved By: Manager of Validation:		Date:

Form Number: V004 (5/28/98)   Reference: SOP-VAL004

See Chapter 6 under "Validation Baseline Document" for information on how to develop and use a validation baseline document.

℞	**Validation Baseline Document**	
Protocol No.: Title:		VBD No.:
Manufacturer:		Page:
Model Number:	Serial Number:	
Equipment Number:	Location:	
Prepared By:		
Validation:		Date:
Approved By:		
Validation Manager:		Date:
Research & Development:		Date:
Operations:		Date:
Maintenance:		Date:
Regulatory Compliance:		Date:

Form Number: V005 (5/28/98)   Page 1 of 2   Reference: SOP-VAL005

Rx	Validation Baseline Document		
Protocol No.:		VBD No.:	
Title:		Page:	
Document Number	Description		Release Date

Form Number: V005 (5/28/98)   Page 2 of 2   Reference: SOP-VAL005

See Chapter 6 under "Validation Change Request Form" for information on how to develop and use a validation change request form.

℞	**Validation Change Request Form**		
Originator:	Date:		VCRF No.:

Validation Baseline Affected: □ Cleaning □ Facility □ Utility □ Equipment □ Computer □ Software □ Process □ Requal	Priority: □ Routine □ Urgent

Documents Affected:		
Document Number	Revision	Title

Reason and Description of Change or (See marked-up documents):

Corrective Action:

Approved By:	
Validation Manager:	Date:
Research & Development:	Date:
Operations:	Date:
Maintenance:	Date:
Regulatory Compliance:	Date:

Form Number: V006 (5/28/98)   Reference: SOP-VAL006

See Chapter 6 under "Deficiency Form" for information on how to develop and use a deficiency form.

℞	**Deficiency Form**		
Prepared by:		Date:	DF No.:
System No.:	Title:		
The deficiency is: Non-Critical ❑ Critical ❑			
Affected Dept(s).:			
Describe the Deficiency:			
Describe the impact if this deficiency is not corrected:			
Correction Action:			
Approved By:			
Validation Manager:			Date:
Maintenance:			Date:

Form Number: V007 (5/28/98)   Reference: SOP-VAL007

See Chapter 8 under "Protocol Package Contents Sheet" for information on how to develop and use a protocol package contents sheet.

℞	**Protocol Package Contents Sheet**			
Equipment Name:				
Equipment No.:	**Model No.:**	**Serial No.:**	**Included:**	
Number	**Description**		**Yes**	**No**

Form Number: V008 (5/28/98)   Reference: SOP-VAL008

Appendix H

Abbreviations

A, Amp	ampere
AC	alternating current
AQL	acceptable quality level
°C	degrees Celsius
cap/hr	capsules per hour
cc	cubic centimeter
cfm	cubic feet per minute
cGMP	Current Good Manufacturing Practices
cm	centimeter
Dia.	diameter
°F	degrees Fahrenheit
FW	final weight
g	gram
GMP	Good Manufacturing Practices
hp	horsepower
hr	hour
Hz	hertz
H_2O	water
in.	inch
in-lb	inch-pounds
in. W.C.	inches water column
IQ	installation qualification
IW	initial weight
kg	kilogram
L	liter
lbs.	pounds
LED	light emitting diode
LOD	loss on drying

min.	minute
mg	milligram
mL	milliliter
mm	millimeter
mm/ss	minutes/seconds
OQ	operational qualification
P&ID	piping and instrumentation diagram
PC	personal computer
PLC	programmable logic controller
PQ	performance qualification
psig	pounds per square inch gauge
rpm	revolutions per minute
Sc	Strongcobb units
sec.	second
SOP	standard operating procedure
TCW	thermal couple wires
tpm	tablets per minute
V	voltage
W.C.	water column

Appendix I

Glossary

Addendum: Additional testing added to a qualification protocol.

Attachment: Supplementary data added to a protocol.

Black Box Software Testing: Evaluates the microprocessor system against the documented functional requirements or intended uses of the system.

Certification: A written approval that a process or system has successfully met all of its defined requirements for validation and can be put into operation.

Deficiency: A problem with a system during qualification testing.

Deviation: A problem with the protocol during qualification testing.

Final Report: A report designed to condense the data generated during the execution of the IQ, OQ, and PQ; contains the results of the overall testing, concludes the results of the data, and also outlines deficiencies and deviations.

Installation Qualification: Documented verification that the equipment is installed in a proper way and that all of the components are installed in an environment suitable for their intended use.

Operational Qualification: Documented verification that the equipment performs as expected throughout its entire operating ranges.

Performance Qualification: Documented verification that the equipment demonstrates effectiveness and repeatability and consistently produces an acceptable product.

Protocol: A written procedure stating how validation will be conducted, including test parameters, production equipment, and decision points on what constitutes acceptable test results; used to document the qualification testing of processing equipment.

Qualification: A process used to determine whether the equipment operates as it was designed to in a reproducible manner.

Revalidation: Reperformance of the validation process or a specific portion thereof.

Validation: Established documented evidence that provides a high degree of assurance that equipment will consistently produce a product meeting its predetermined specifications and quality attributes.

Appendix J

Recommended Reading

Baker, G. S. and Rhodes, C. T. 1996. *Modern Pharmaceutics*. New York: Marcel Dekker, Inc.

Berry, I. R. and Harpaz, D. 1997. *Validation of Bulk Pharmaceutical Chemicals*. Buffalo Grove: Interpharm Press, Inc.

Berry, I. R. and Nash, R. A. 1993. *Pharmaceutical Process Validation*. New York: Marcel Dekker, Inc.

DeSain, C. 1993a. *Documentation Basics that Support Good Manufacturing Practices*. Buffalo Grove: Interpharm Press, Inc.

DeSain, C. 1993b. *Drug Device and Diagnostic Manufacturing*. Buffalo Grove: Interpharm Press, Inc.

DeSain, C. V. and Sutton, C. V. 1997. *Validation for Medical Device and Diagnostic Manufacturers*. Buffalo Grove: Interpharm Press, Inc.

Juran, J. M. and Gryna, F. M. 1988. *Juran's Quality Control Handbook*. New York: McGraw-Hill, Inc.

Lachman, L., Lieberman, H. A. and Kanig, J. L. 1986. *The Theory and Practice of Industrial Pharmacy*. Philadelphia: Lea & Febiger.

Stokes, T., Branning, R. C., Chapman, K. G., Hamblock, H. and Trill, A. J. 1994. *Good Computer Validation Practices*. Buffalo Grove: Interpharm Press, Inc.

Willing, S. H. and Stoker, J. R. 1992. *Good Manufacturing Practices for Pharmaceuticals*. New York: Marcel Dekker, Inc.

Wingate, G. 1997 *Validating Automated Manufacturing and Laboratory Applications*. Buffalo Grove: Interpharm Press, Inc.

Index